CW00468392

BREAST CANCER

A journey from fear to empowerment

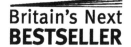

Britain's Next
BESTSELLER

First published in 2014 by:

Britain's Next Bestseller
An imprint of Live It Publishing
27 Old Gloucester Road
London, United Kingdom.
WC1N 3AX

www.britainsnextbestseller.co.uk

Copyright © 2014 by Cath Filby

The moral right of Cath Filby to be identified as the author
of this work has been asserted by her in accordance with the
Copyright, Designs and Patents Act 1988.

All rights reserved.

Except as permitted under current legislation, no part of this
work may be photocopied, stored in a retrieval system,
published, performed in public, adapted, broadcast, transmitted,
recorded or reproduced in any form or by any means, without
the prior permission of the copyright owners.

All enquiries should be addressed to Britain's Next Bestseller.

ISBN 978-1-906954-89-5 (pbk)

DEDICATION

This book is dedicated to all of the women who have already taken, or may, in the future, find themselves taking, the journey through cancer. I hope that you will find my personal experience and this self-help method of approach motivating, help you deal with any fears you may experience on your journey and that you will discover how empowering it is to take control of your health.

God Bless and Good Luck.

ACKNOWLEDGEMENTS

I acknowledge with love and gratitude the following people:

My amazing husband, whose strength during our darkest moments together never ceased to surprise me.

My eldest son, John, whose memory continues to teach me how to be strong and who fills my life with so much love that I could burst.

My other two remarkable children, Paula and Richard Jnr, who demonstrated during my illness what compassionate, mature and caring people they have become. I am so proud and humbled to have them in my life.

Our first grandchild, Louis-John, whose smile and funny little ways filled my thoughts and helped me through the long black nights when I couldn't sleep. Our first granddaughter, Mariella, who, like her brother, is such a joy and adds to my reason for being. Their father Jon, who offered words of wisdom to me and great understanding and support to my daughter during a very difficult period in her life.

My wonderful daughter-in-law, Milla, and my two other beautiful grand-daughters, Nancy and Molly, who contribute such fun and laughter to our family.

My mother, whose philosophy and mothering skills have been an inspiration to me throughout my life.

My Godson, Oliver, who, through his untimely death,

showed me the real importance of being in, and cherishing, the moment.

Dr Emilio Alba and his Oncology team at the Clinica CROASA Radioterapia y Oncología in Malaga, Spain, who provided me at all times with support, reassurance and the benefit of their great medical expertise.

All of the personnel that I encountered when following the complementary therapy path: Bill and Jennifer from the Health Centre 'Cause and Effect' in Sevierville, Tennessee; Kevin Day, of Las Mariposas Clinic in Fuengirola, Malaga, Spain, and anyone else who advised me on supplements and treatments. Their expertise was much appreciated.

Lynne Sherratt, who was responsible for putting me in touch with the breast reconstruction technique that was to change my life. Many thanks, Lynne, and keep devouring all that knowledge!

Ms Elaine Sassoon and her team of professionals who, with their amazing skills, performed a physical miracle on me. Keep up the great work.

The Exeter Friendly Society Private Medical Insurance Company, who delivered a very professional and supportive service during my cancer treatment and reconstruction procedures.

Murielle Maupoint, from Live It Publishing, and the Britain's Next Best Seller team, who believed in my book's potential to get my message out there and who supported me through my steep Social Networking learning curve.

And, last but not least, the rest of our family and good friends cannot go unmentioned because, without them, my journey would have been far harder. Their abundant love, humour, practical gifts and soup were received with much gratitude!

Thank you to all the people
who made this book possible...

Elaine Hargrove, Oli Smith, Darren Sayers, Ema Hamlin,
Oliver Smith, Richard Filby, Kat Zoula, Camilla Filby,
Laura Slater, Ellen Murray, Ema Hamlin, Claire Hocking,
Gemma Burden, Kate Pinnuck, Saskia Stephenson,
Shirley Anne Norminton, Jon, Paula, Louis-John, Mariella,
Sally Hay, Jenny Sargent, Adele-Marie,
Liz Fathers, Becky Armstrong, Tina Barton, Debbie Birch,
Michelle Needham, Sasha Stockley, Liz Dean, Mike Dean,
Chantelle Dean, David Foster, Joanna Gasiorowska,
Lynne and Brian Sherratt, Dee and Robert Pollard,
Alexandra Burton, Maeve Carroll, Annie, Jose Stracke,
Janice Fitzgerald, Kathryn Diver, Eric Shaw, Florence,
Jan Freegard, Breast Cancer CARE WA, Eli Medalen,
Kerry Schreier, Vicki O'Raw, Gemma Easthope,
Sonia Dutton, Jodie Carla Smith, My Absolute Image,
Sherry Marlow, Joanna Alsford, Kate Pinnuck,
Margaret & Ken Calkin, Jeannie Bucci, Ryan Mark,
Jane McCormack, Muriel Lundy, Matt Gugiatti,
Llinos Thomas, Valerie Ducie, Clare E Hawkins,
David Smith, Karen Bavastock, Nina Sollitt, Joan Bithell,
Paula Mouret-Lafage, Luisa Camacho.

*And to everyone else who chose to
remain anonymous...*

CONTENTS

FOREWORD

AS I commence typing the first part of my self-help book, my mind is full of so many ideas, thoughts and experiences that I must share with you, the reader. I realize how important it is that this book fulfils its main objective: to offer a practical guide to anyone who follows the journey through cancer, hoping that it will free you from the fear of this terrible disease and give you the understanding that you have the power to aid your recovery.

On diagnosis, I know how important it is to find some help and information quickly. Taking back control of your mind as it is invaded with irrational thoughts and unreasonable emotions and preventing it from descending into an abyss of despair must become a priority. I discovered that focusing on improving my health through a structured healthy-living plan and re-arming my natural defence mechanism was extremely motivating. This approach also provided an invaluable overall feeling of well-being at a time when my body was about to reach its lowest ebb.

An understandable reaction is to demand some answers to questions like *why?* and *how?* Unfortunately, there is not just one answer to one question and, because everyone is so unique, every individual's questions will be different. Often when answers are not forthcoming, one's immediate reaction is to panic. However, in the first part of this book, I intend to outline my own story and personal experience, hoping that it will offer some insight into what a unique journey is ahead; how, because cancer is so full of paradoxes, there are benefits and humour to be found in the most unlikely circumstances; and how, if we really want to, we can grow as individuals as a result of what may seem at the time, one of life's cruellest blows.

CHAPTER 1

UNBELIEVABLE

'A young pedestrian was knocked down whilst walking along the Newtown to Kerry road at 8.10 p.m., this evening.'

After all these years I can still remember those words as if it was yesterday and this is where, I believe, my journey through cancer began. On November 8th 1990, at approximately 9.50 pm, two rather burly-looking policemen had appeared at the door of our idyllic country cottage in the heart of Mid-Wales, Powys, UK.

At first, I was afraid to invite them in, for fear of what further bad news they were likely to convey. Then, suddenly, as if remembering my manners and feeling sorry that they had been given the task of delivering such bad news, I went into autopilot and invited them to cross the threshold into our kitchen-diner. At that moment our daughter, Paula, appeared, curious to know why there were policeman in her home. Knowing instinctively that there was more bad news to come, I asked her to make a cup of tea and ushered the visitors into another room.

They refused my offer to sit down and, before they could say any more, I asked if the pedestrian was badly hurt.

It was then that I noticed that one of them was carrying our seventeen year-old son, John's, rucksack. When they handed me his newly-acquired driving licence and the Edinburgh Fringe Festival Identity Card that he always carried in his wallet, and by the look on their faces, I knew he was dead. One of them verbally confirmed this, explaining that John had been struck from behind by a high-powered motorcycle. By now, my autopilot had taken full control, and still feeling extremely sorry for them, I offered them a cup of tea, which they declined.

My next thought was to explain to Paula as quickly as possible that John had died and called her into the lounge to break the shattering news. Months later, I watched a TV documentary on the subject of grief, which stated that, if a child loses a close relative, you must always communicate the truth as soon as possible following the death. I didn't know this at the time.

Shattering it was, for us both, and we clung on to each other for what seemed like an eternity. Paula and John were extremely close and she idolised her elder brother. For many months following his death, she carried out her studies and lived her life as a robot, hardly able to mention his name. She was only fourteen years old.

My husband, Richard, who was at a football meeting that evening, later told me that, on hearing the news to go home, he instinctively felt that something had happened to one of the children. One can only imagine what a dreadful journey it was for him as he drove home that cold, dark November night.

Our nine year old younger son, Richard jnr., dealt with John's death very differently and demonstrated what we thought at the time was extremely sensitive behaviour that belied his years. He always seemed to be available to comfort and console us when the need arose and our tears flowed uncontrollably in the early weeks following John's death. His gentle support was especially appreciated by his father, who sought and found great comfort from his little son's loving ways and they would often be found, on the settee, huddled together, their arms wrapped around one another.

Little had we realized, during this time, was that young Richard was actually seeking out comfort from us for his own grief at losing his brother. Cocooned in our own painful feelings, we missed the signals of cries for help coming from this little boy. Knowing what I know now, as his mother, I certainly would not have shut down and cloaked myself in what felt like armour plate to bury the pain I was experiencing. My father had died of lung cancer three months earlier and I never did grieve properly for him. His death seemed to pale into insignificance compared to the agony I and my family were feeling at the loss of our John.

During the early years, following his death, I would suggest to the rest of my nuclear family that perhaps we should go to family bereavement counselling, wondering if this would help us to understand what effect John's death was having on us as a family. The rest of the family never did take up my offer and, on reflection, I realised that we were all at different stages of the grieving process, unable to bear our own pain, let alone one another's.

Although, over the next few months following the funeral, individual counselling was given to our daughter, my husband and myself, young Richard chose to go much later, when he was twenty three years old and had hit a

3

difficult period in his life. We will never know whether group counselling would have helped us deal with the trauma more effectively as a family.

The wisdom of hindsight is an amazing concept and the reflection I have of this stage of my journey shows me that the coping strategies I demonstrated at times certainly did not offer the best solution for me or my family. One such coping strategy was returning to work, two weeks after John's death. Our business became a welcome relief and distraction although, looking back, Richard and I both say that much of the enthusiasm and motivation for the business left us after John died and it never quite had the same meaning, somehow. To outsiders, we coped with the loss of our eldest son and got on with our lives for the sake of our remaining two children, the rest of our extended families and one another.

Often, people would remark how wonderfully I had coped and, looking back, it was not so much a brave face as the fear of staying in the abyss I had found myself in during the days following John's death. I knew that, at the young age of thirty five, I did not want to remain in a black hole for ever. 'Life goes on' - a phrase which would become my mantra for years to come, and to my detriment.

The death of a popular young man in his prime affects a wide circle of people and, as we have a large extended family, there was a lot of heartbreak to deal with. Without our wonderful family and friends, I don't know how we would have survived the dark days. My elder sister was an angel and, despite having to deal with her own heartbreak at losing her nephew, who was also her godson, she seemed to offer us the strength and faith that one day we would see John again.

My mother quietly supported us, as was her way, by looking after Richard Jnr when we were working, and by listening to our anxieties when necessary. When mother wasn't around, a dear friend, who is the mother of my best school friend and who I have known since I was four, would offer support and a shoulder to cry on. What would we have done without these exceptional people and their help? Little did I know that a similar tragic story would happen some sixteen years later and I would find myself in the same situation as our family and friends had found themselves in when John died.

The following years proved extremely fruitful with the growth of our business. Gaining national success as a quality organisation allowed us to eventually sell the business and retire to Spain when we were still in our forties. As with all owner-managed businesses, there had been a price to pay for the success and it came in the guise of a lot of very hard work, accompanied by a great deal of stress. One thing is for certain: for both of us, our business was very much a means of escape from our shared grief.

Fortunately, apart from the usual teenage issues, Paula and Richard Jnr got on with their lives, maturing into loving, successful adults and, as a family, we have developed extremely rewarding relationships with one another. That isn't to say that we have really ever fully recovered from John's death and an event in January 2006 proved to me that I was never far from the edge of that deep void I had experienced late in 1990.

Our retirement to Spain was a real tonic for rebuilding our life and allowed us to take it in a new direction, forming wonderful friendships, experiencing a new culture and masking some of the pain. The children were settled in their chosen careers in the UK and seemed pleased about the prospect of visiting us in Spain when the opportunity arose. We had bought a large family villa and had visions of enjoying many quality times together, relaxing around the swimming pool and chatting over long lunches on the sun terrace - and this we certainly did.

The next ten years passed relatively uneventfully with the usual family events of births, weddings and the funerals of elderly relatives. The worst problem that occurred was that Richard had a rather serious back operation, brought on from all the renovation work in our homes that he had carried out during our 38 years of marriage. Thankfully, he recovered extremely well and continues with his running, completing the 2008 London Marathon for the Breast Cancer Care charity in just less than four and a half hours.

CHAPTER 2

THE PRE-CANCEROUS YEARS

IF you believe, as I do, that everything that happens in our lives physically and emotionally leaves an imprint on our mind and body, I should include my formative years as well as the events leading up to my diagnosis, in describing my journey through cancer. I wasn't keen to do this as I didn't want to travel down any slip roads at this stage of the journey and deflect from the real issue at hand, the sharing of my journey through cancer.

My daughter often says that she doesn't know how my siblings and I came through such a traumatic childhood so unscathed. The fact that my brother, two sisters and I managed to create relatively successful lives for ourselves was due, in part, to the stoical and strong mother we had, the middle-class town we lived in, the state schools that we attended, the friends we made and, in my case, the marriage partner I found at the age of fifteen.

Yes, life could have been better when we were growing up. To have a violent, alcoholic father, who spent most of his wages every week gambling was not a good way to start one's journey through life.

However, that is one part of my life journey that I have reconciled by understanding that out of those traumatic times evolved an understanding of how important it is to try to come to terms with your own life circumstances and learn as much as you can from them. It created in me an emotional sensitivity and empathy for anyone who was suffering a trauma in their life and a desire to comfort those who demonstrated a degree of vulnerability or sadness. It certainly taught me that no matter how much I loved my man, he would not treat me the way my mother was treated in her marriage.

As well as the close relationship I had with my mother and siblings, when I was growing up, I was also fortunate to have a few other people who had a profound effect on my views and values and helped to mould me into the person I am today. The teaching staff at my Church of England primary school were responsible for giving me grounding in a religious faith, which has, through my life experiences to date, enabled me to find a God I am comfortable with.

It was during my primary school years, which, in the 1950s, one started very early (I was just four years old), that I was to meet my best school friend, Paula (yes, we named our daughter after her). She would prove to be a loyal, sensitive and generous companion who would accompany me to Secondary school, be Godmother to my daughter and who would always remain, over the coming years, somewhere in the background of my life.

Although we had spent many school years together, sharing adolescent problems, the same sense of humour and life values, we didn't see one another regularly when she moved to Paris to become a fashion model. There she remained, marrying a Frenchman and raising a charming, handsome son. Fortunately, during my childhood, I formed a very close bond with her mother and father and they became surrogate grandparents to our grandchildren, eventually moving to Wales to be close to us. They, with my mother, proved at times to be our salvation, providing the extended family network that was much needed during those early years when our business was growing and we were all trying to cope with the loss of John.

Paula and I kept in touch mainly through her parents and she knew that, as they moved into retirement, we would always look after them if they needed help, now and then. I became Godmother to her son, Oliver, and I had followed his progress closely during the first twenty-one years of his life, spending time with him when he came to Wales for long vacations with his grandparents or when we visited France. We spoke on the telephone when it was his birthday and at Christmas, and he had visited us in Spain. When we met up with him in 2005 for his grandmother's eightieth birthday, I was delighted to see how he had grown into a funny, sensitive and beautiful young man, who adored his parents.

I made sure I telephoned him that year, when he was in the South of France where he was working, for his twenty-first birthday and, the same year, we spoke on Boxing Day, when he explained, excitedly, that he was off to Morocco with some friends for the New Year celebrations. I remember specifically asking, as I would my own children, if it was safe over there and to take care. He assured me that it was perfectly safe, not to worry and that he would have great time. What happened next proved unbelievable and I still have trouble coming to terms with it.

A week after I spoke to Oliver, we received a 'phone call from his mother, telling us that Oliver and two other friends had died in an accident in the house where they

9

were staying in Morocco. All I can remember is screaming and sobbing in disbelief that this had happened to my best friend. What was even more tragic was that he was her only child - such a beautiful son and taken, like our John, so tragically.

The days, weeks and months that followed were unimaginably painful for the family. As Paula and her husband had to remain in France, trying to unravel the events surrounding their son's death, it fell to us to break the news to his elderly grandparents. This was as distressing as when I heard the news about losing our son.

We did what we could to support Paula, her husband, Joël, and her parents and, overnight, Paula and I rekindled the closeness we had nurtured in childhood, the deaths of our sons bonding us together in unlikely, unbelievable circumstances.

I tried to support with words of empathy, knowing full well what she was going through as a mother, and offered advice if I thought it would help. Many times, I referred back to my own and my family's experience when she asked me questions about how I had coped.

It is now eight years since Oliver died, and Paula and Joël are trying to get on with their lives without their son, and I know that they have their good days as well as their bad ones. I also know that, during the good days, they may experience unexpected moments when a word, a piece of music, a rendezvous with a friend or anniversaries will send them immediately into a downward spiral. What I don't know and can only imagine is what it is like to lose an only child.

For me, losing my godson compared greatly with losing

my own son and, during the six months following Oliver's death, I remember that all my motivation for life drained away. Everything seemed pointless and my faith was truly tested. Looking back, I realise that I sank into a kind of depression, which saw me functioning physically on a daily basis but, emotionally and spiritually, I was not coping at all.

Not even the birth of my first grandchild, in April 2007, jogged me out of my grieving despair. What made it worse was that I didn't know that this was happening to me, although I know that it was really difficult to speak with anyone and, often, I was just going through the motions of polite conversation. I never felt unable to talk with Paula and many hours were spent on the 'phone together, going over the same question that I had asked that November night in 1990 when John died: "Why?"

Some might say that we were being self-indulgent or self-piteous in our grief. Well, I would say to those people that the talking and analysing helps and, although you never discover the answer to your questions, sharing one's grief is comforting and a gentle tonic that alleviates the pain for a short time.

Today, the numbness has subsided and my zest for life has returned as a result, ironically enough, of my diagnosis for breast cancer. I still have days or moments when I am extremely sad over the loss of Oliver as I am about losing my own son. I try to remember my own philosophy that helped me during the initial grief for John: it is better to have had them for their short time on Earth than never to have had them in my life at all. I was privileged to have seen them both grow into handsome, sensitive and affectionate young men. It helps to imagine that John and Oliver may be angels in Heaven, together.

However, the pain I feel for my dear friend pulls constantly at my heart and I have wished many times for a way to ease the hurt that I know she feels, or take it away from her completely. It is so cruel and quite extraordinary to think that fate has dealt us both the same hand! Although time seems to stop when you suffer such a massive blow in your life, life really does go on and, somehow, we all picked up the pieces after Oliver died and destiny led me towards another of life's extraordinary journeys.

Although I believe that fate plays a role in our life, how we deal with our destiny is within our control. During my search for some answers as to why I, of all people, should have contracted cancer, I looked at the usual well-documented lifestyle factors as possible causes such as hereditary links, bad diet, too much alcohol, inadequate exercise, smoking, environmental factors and stress. I came to the conclusion that the only one that may be relevant was stress and, even taking this factor into my health equation, I thought that I had always coped quite well with stressful situations.

I had always encouraged us to have a healthy lifestyle, I had breast-fed all of my children, only drank alcohol on social occasions and I had my ovaries removed during a hysterectomy when I was forty-three. So, in theory, my oestrogen levels should have been lower than normal, although this did throw me into a pre-menopausal state very early. Within the masses of resources I was accumulating, I came across an interesting article on the internet which gave me an insight into the massive impact losing my son and godson may have had on my long term health:

1. *"On August 18, 1978, Dr. Ryke Geerd Hamer, M.D., at the time head internist in the oncology clinic at the University of Munich, Germany, received the shocking news*

that his son Dirk had been shot. Dirk died in December 1978. A few months later, Dr. Hamer was diagnosed with testicular cancer. Since he had never been seriously ill, he immediately surmised that his cancer development might be directly related to the tragic loss of his son. Dirk's death and his own experience with cancer prompted Dr. Hamer to investigate the personal history of his cancer patients. He quickly learned that, like him, they all had gone through some exceptionally stressful episode prior to developing cancer. The observation of a mind-body connection was not really surprising. Numerous studies had already shown that cancer and other diseases are often preceded by a traumatic event. However, Dr. Hamer took his research a momentous step further and pursued the hypothesis that all bodily events are controlled from the brain. He analyzed his patients' brain scans and compared them with their medical records and discovered that every disease — not only cancer! — is controlled from its own specific area in the brain and linked to a very particular, identifiable, "conflict shock". The result of his research is a scientific chart that illustrates the biological relationship between the psyche and the brain in correlation with the organs and tissues of the entire human body.

Dr. Hamer came to call his findings **"The Five Biological Laws of the New Medicine"**, because these biological laws, which are applicable to any patient's case, offer an entirely new understanding of the cause, the development, and the natural healing process of diseases. (In response to the growing number of misrepresentations of his discoveries and to preserve the integrity and authenticity of his scientific work, Dr. Hamer has now legally protected his research material under the name German New Medicine® (GNM). The term "New Medicine" cannot be copyrighted internationally.

13

In 1981, Dr. Hamer presented his findings to the Medical Faculty of the University of Tübingen as a post-doctoral thesis. But to this day, the University has refused to test Dr. Hamer's research in spite of its legal obligation to do so. This is an unprecedented case in the history of universities. Similarly, official medicine refuses to approve his discoveries despite some 30 scientific verifications both by independent physicians and by professional associations.

Shortly after Dr. Hamer submitted his thesis, he was given the ultimatum to renounce his discoveries or have his contract renewal at the University clinic denied. In 1986, even though his scientific work had never been impeached, much less disproved, Dr. Hamer was stripped of his medical license on the grounds that he refused to conform to the principles of standard medicine. Yet he was determined to continue his work. By 1987 he was able to extend his discoveries to practically every disease known to medicine.

Dr. Hamer has been persecuted and harassed for over 25 years, in particular by the German and French authorities and since 1997 he has been living in exile in Spain, where he carries on with his research and where he continues to fight for official recognition of his "New Medicine". As long as the University of Tübingen's medical faculty maintains its delay tactics, patients all over the world will be denied the benefit of Dr. Hamer's revolutionary discoveries.

Dr. Hamer established that "every disease is caused by a conflict shock that catches an individual completely off guard" (First Biological Law). In honour of his son, this unanticipated stressful event has been called a Dirk Hamer Syndrome or DHS. Psychologically speaking, a DHS is a very personal incident conditioned by our past experiences, our vulnerabilities, our individual perceptions, our values and beliefs. Yet, a DHS is not merely a psychological but

14

rather a biological conflict that has to be understood in the context of our evolution.

Animals experience these biological shocks in concrete terms, for example through a sudden loss of the nest or territory, a loss of an offspring, a separation from a mate or from the pack, an unexpected threat of starvation, or a death-fright. Since, over time, the human mind acquired a figurative way of thinking, we can experience these biological conflicts also in a transposed sense. A male, for instance, can suffer a "territorial loss conflict" when he unexpectedly loses his home or his workplace; a female "nest conflict" may be a concern over the well-being of a "nest member"; an "abandonment conflict" can be triggered by an unforeseen divorce or, by being rushed to hospital, children often suffer a "separation conflict".

By analyzing thousands of brain computer tomograms (CT) in relation to his patients' histories, Dr. Hamer discovered that the moment a DHS occurs, the shock impacts a specific, predetermined area in the brain, causing a "lesion" that is visible on a CT scan as a set of sharp concentric rings (In 1989, Siemens, the German CT scanner manufacturer, certified that these ring formations are not errors in the functioning of the equipment). Upon impact, the affected brain cells communicate the shock to the corresponding organ, which in turn responds with a particular predictable alteration. The reason why specific conflicts are indissolubly tied to specific brain areas is that during our historical evolution, each part of the brain was programmed to respond instantly to conflicts that could threaten our survival. While the "old brain" (brain stem and cerebellum) is programmed with basic survival issues that relate to breathing, eating or reproduction, the "new brain" (cerebrum) is encoded with more advanced themes such

15

as territorial conflicts, separation conflicts, identity conflicts, and self-devaluation conflicts.'

To summarise, the German New Medicine (GNM) operates under the premise that every disease, including cancer, originates from an unexpected shock experience. If the shock catches an individual completely off-guard, provided there is a resolution of the conflict, every disease proceeds in two phases, a conflict-active phase and a healing phase. *'Every so-called disease has to be understood as a meaningful special biological program of nature created to solve an unexpected biological conflict.'* If someone dies (the conflict-active phase of the disease), it is believed to be *'because of energy loss, weight loss, sleep deprivation, emotional and mental exhaustion. The stress of receiving a cancer diagnosis, or being given a negative prognosis, is often enough to deprive a person of their life-force.'*

I most certainly agree with the final point as my immediate reaction to my biopsy result was that I was going to die. However, whether it was instinct, faith, love from my family, or all three, I soon realised that negative thoughts were sending me on a downward spiral and I knew I would need to be as focused as possible on staying positive.

A philosophy I read during my research into cures for cancer that makes such sense is called 'inverse paranoid'. American billionaire and philanthropist, W. Clement Stone (who, coincidentally, had a father who left his family impoverished due to his gambling addiction), firmly believed that most of the negative events that occur in our lives can be turned around into positives and viewed as lessons, ultimately improving our characters in someway: "Like success, failure is many things to many people. With Positive Mental Attitude, failure is a learning experience, a rung on the ladder, and a plateau at which to get your thoughts in order and prepare to try again." Well, I was certainly determined, during my journey, to learn some constructive lessons from this latest experience, and to improve myself and my lifestyle.

I now believe that all of my experiences throughout my life to date have had a cause and effect on my health, primarily in the way that I have dealt with these life experiences. Before I was diagnosed with cancer, I had not appreciated how seriously stress could damage your health and, more importantly, your immune system. Since my hysterectomy when I was forty-three, I had had a fear of putting on weight and I always tried to maintain a consistent exercise routine, running on average three times a week. I have always enjoyed good food and believed that I ate a healthy, balanced diet. Therefore, what could have gone wrong?

As my journey unfolded, the horizon ahead would become clearer and I would discover some answers to the many questions that initially crowded my panicked mind.

The research I was starting to carry out as part of my quest to be free of the cancer was helping me to understand how the traumas that I had suffered - the loss of a child like Dr Hamer and, sixteen years later, the loss of my godson - had had such a profound effect on my health. I began to appreciate that the reason I had cancer was not entirely my fault and my doctor, at the time of my diagnosis, suggested that my current fitness level may have certainly prevented the disease from spreading.

However, the relationship between my physical well being and the birth of my tumour was only part of the story. It was becoming evident that it was not just the stress that causes the distress in your body but also the way you handle that stress/distress. I was starting to really appreciate how it is very important to have an extremely healthy immune system to cope with any disease which may invade the body. Paradoxically, the immune system is greatly affected by stress.

Notes to Chapter 2

1. © By Caroline Markolin, Ph.D., Vancouver, Canada

2. 'Since 1998, Dr. Hamer's discoveries have never been disproved, only criticized as not being in accordance with the common view, i.e. with the theories and hypotheses of standard medicine.

'In view of the German Superior Court verdict (BGH-IV ZR 135/92) that every cancer therapy is in fact an experiment and that standard medicine is unable to understand cancer on a scientific basis, the ongoing suppression of the German New Medicine® and Dr. Hamer's imprisonment seems unfathomable.'

EXPLORE Article - http://LearningGNM.com/documents/gnm_articles___ introduction.html or the pdf version http://LearningGNM.com/documents/ Explore%20Article%20-%20English.pdf

PEN Letter - http://LearningGNM.com/documents/penletter.html or its pdf version http://LearningGNM.com/documents/Penn.pdf

CHAPTER 3

TOO BUSY TO NOTICE

THE first time I knew there was something wrong was early one morning in September 2007 when we were staying with our daughter, having returned suddenly to the UK from our home in Spain for the funeral of Oliver's eighty-eight year old grandfather, Lucas, who had died suddenly.

Richard and I were lying in bed, having woken early after a restless night, and were discussing the arrangements for the day. As our family were very close to Lucas, naturally we were very upset and had offered to help the bereaved family with the funeral arrangements.

As I was lying on my right side with my left hand resting on my right breast, I felt an unusual lump. I must add at this point that as my breasts were only, at most, size 34A, it was easy to detect any abnormal changes. I had suffered with benign breast disease (fibrotic benign breast disease, to be exact) since my late twenties and often discovered benign cysts which I would sometimes have aspirated.

I had had my annual breast check up with my gynae-cologist in Spain in February of that year. Although she had not discovered any abnormalities at the time, she had recommended a mammogram. Unfortunately, because we were moving house and had made rather a lot of plans, such as travelling to the UK to await the birth of our first grandchild, I had decided to wait for my mammogram until we returned to Spain in September.

As I lay there, carrying out my self-examination, I realised that I was not the only one who was an expert on my breasts and turned to my husband, Richard, to ask for a second opinion. His advice was to get it checked out as it seemed rather large and hard.

Events over the next few weeks would delay me booking a check-up still further because, when shortly after we returned to Spain, following Lucas' funeral, another very good friend died and we had to return almost immediately to the UK for yet another funeral.

By the time we returned to Spain and the appointment was finally made with the doctor, it was mid-October. During the examination with the doctor, he drained some fluid from the lump and carried out an ultrasound check. His diagnosis was that he would like me to go to the hospital for a full biopsy.

People ask me if I knew then that it was cancer and, when I look back, deep down, I knew that something was different about this lump but I tried to be positive. I remember feeling tired, and sleeping in the afternoon was not something I was prone to doing.

My Goddaughter and her friend were staying with us for the half-term holiday and this was a welcome relief from the sadness of the previous few weeks and from any concerns we had over the results of the biopsy which were due the following week.

My mantra came to mind: 'life goes on', and it certainly

does, as I was to find out over the next few months. Life goes on around you while you feel that yours has come to a standstill - a little paradox of the journey that was ahead of me. At this point I want to add that although at times you feel that you are a lone traveller, you will find that many people will join you at different times on your journey if you allow them to.

I mentioned that, during the last few months of 2007, life was hectic and November proved to be no exception. We had agreed to house-sit for some friends who had gone on holiday to the UK and we tried to busy ourselves with this distraction while we endured the ten days waiting to receive the results of my biopsy. All sorts of thoughts go through your mind and you oscillate from 'yes, you have breast cancer' to 'don't be so ridiculous, you can't possibly have it!'

I thought that I had always tried very hard to look after myself, eating healthily, not drinking much alcohol and, since my hysterectomy when I was forty-three, I had run, on average, two to three times a week, completing the London Marathon in 2005 on behalf of the Parkinson's Society. I had also breast fed all three of my children - the youngest until he was nine months old - another reason my breasts had shrunk to nothing! As I received my diagnosis I wondered whether I had looked after myself so well after all.

The night before the results, Richard and I did not sleep well and we were very glad when the day finally arrived to discover the outcome of the biopsy. We collected the results from the hospital and then had to travel to another clinic for my appointment with my doctor. The private health care system in Spain has a very relaxed approach and, as the results were handed to me in an unsealed envelope, I knew that the doctor would not worry if I opened it.

I couldn't wait to get out of the hospital to read the diagnosis. Standing in front of the hospital entrance, I ripped open the envelope. Naturally, the diagnosis was in Spanish but the Latin terminology for cancer was very recognisable in Spanish: carcinoma ductal. The words hit me right in the pit of my stomach and my hands shook as I showed Richard the results. Before he had a chance to read them properly, I ran up to two Spanish nurses who were leaving the hospital, waving my results under their noses, and asked them to translate the diagnosis for me. Naturally, they declined and told me to see my doctor.

At that stage the numbness had started to set in and, looking at Richard's face, I knew he feared the worst, like I did: that I was going to die. The journey to the clinic and the final wait in the reception area before we were called in to see the doctor seemed to last an eternity. We just wanted confirmation of how bad things were and what the outcome was likely to be.

Although Richard and I are never short of conversation - at least, I am certainly not - we hardly spoke during this time. We didn't really need to say much as we both knew that, whatever the outcome of the biopsy, we were on this journey together. That's how it had always been during our marriage. Whenever there was a predicament or problem to solve, we found a solution and discussed the way forward.

When we were partners in our business, staff were always amazed at how professionally we conducted ourselves, never arguing or undermining one another. That isn't to say that we don't argue and still do have our humdingers (ask our children!), mainly due to my headstrong, stubborn streak. Somehow, though, we have always worked together and stand united in a crisis and this crisis was going to be no different.

During the first appointment, the doctor explained in broken English and some Spanish that the biopsy had shown a lump of approximately three centimetres in size in the upper pole of my right breast. He could not say what type of cancer it was (at this stage I did not realise that there was more than one type of breast cancer) and he recommended a lumpectomy and any further treatment would depend on the type of cancer and whether it had spread. Removal of some of my lymph nodes would be a possibility and he would know more when I was on the operating table. He offered to carry out the operation that very week, within the following two days.

Sitting opposite the doctor, I felt a hot glow creeping slowly throughout my body. This menopausal hot flush gathered pace as it travelled towards my head and I felt as though I was going to explode with the panic that had taken over my body. I wanted to shout at the doctor, 'Hang on a minute. I need time to take stock and decide what exactly I want done to my body!' Fortunately, my rational self kicked in and many questions started to formulate in my head as the hot flush quickly subsided.

My first question was, 'What is the likelihood of the cancer returning or spreading to the other breast?' Under the circumstances, this was a perfectly natural question and I just wanted him to reassure me, there and then, that, once he had cut out the lump, there was a 100 per cent guarantee that it would not return.

A natural question it may be but a stupid one also,

as no competent surgeon is going to give their patient a cast iron guarantee that carrying out a lumpectomy will be the end of the situation. Reading between the lines of his response, it was becoming evident that there was another option open to me. A full mastectomy was looking like a realistic alternative. Mainly because of the condition of my left breast, which had had a rather large mass of cysts removed eighteen years previously and, with the possibility of further cysts or tumours occurring in either breast, I started seriously to consider removal of both breasts.

During the silence that followed, I quietly explained my thoughts to Richard and, seeing no immediate response in his eyes either way, I put forward the possibility to the surgeon opposite, asking again whether this would give me the protection from the cancer recurring in the future. His response was as positive as he dared communicate and I felt that it may improve my chances of long term survival. He also added that the chemotherapy, if I had to have a course, and taking an oestrogen inhibiting drug called Tamoxifen for five years would considerably increase the likelihood of the cancer staying in remission.

At that stage, I knew very little about breast cancer, only superficial information that you find in women's magazines. However, I always seemed to be hearing of women with breast cancer who had had a lumpectomy and then had to return to the operating table for a mastectomy. I could also see before me years of worry for Richard and me, every time a cyst appeared or I felt a protrusion in either breast. I was not relishing the thought of losing my breasts and, had it been the left breast that was cancerous, I think I would have thought twice about a bi-lateral mastectomy, because my right breast would have been worth saving. However, there wasn't much left of the left breast so I needed to go away and give serious consideration to the type of operation I was going to have.

I want to say at this point to all of the readers of this book that in no way am I advocating having a mastectomy in preference to a lumpectomy. Every woman's medical situation is unique and it is extremely important that you take as much information and advice from the medical experts to enable you to make an informed decision.

A variety of people have since spoken to me about the reasoning behind the decision I made to remove my breasts. Many have asked me if, in hindsight, I would have taken a different path of treatment. For me, the path I chose was correct because it gave me the opportunity to take control of my situation and not let it control me too much - an important point when you are looking to draw on all your reserves of strength to fight what is ahead.

In those first few days and weeks, the reaction I was experiencing was a loss of self-esteem as the horror of what I perceived lay ahead: the inability to make future plans, the removal of my breasts, and the possible demise of my body. The perception of loss of any control I might have had over my life overwhelmed me. You are right to sense that I am a person who likes to be in control as opposed to controlling, and there is a subtle difference. I have always enjoyed being proactive and making things happen whether that is in my professional life, my family life or my social life.

The maintenance of my own and my family's health was not excluded from the tenacious way in which I had organised our life. I firmly believed, and still do, that we have a role to play in the management of our well-being and good health. Therefore, when I was struck down with cancer at the age of fifty-three, the shock was a severe blow to my perception, at that time, of how well I had managed my life.

Suddenly I was thrown into a pool of instant decision-making with any time for reflection not an option. I felt that time was not on my side. I have since learnt that a little extra time was something I certainly did have on my side and I would urge anyone who is given a diagnosis of cancer to step back and think through the options and what complementary approaches are available to you.

You must talk to other doctors about your prognosis as this proved to be one way I felt I was able to take back a little control over my body and my life and try to restore the self-confidence I had suddenly lost.

I returned to the UK for a second opinion and a private consultation with a breast cancer specialist. I also wanted to discover whether it would be advantageous to return to my homeland and have my operation there. I thought, naively, that perhaps a second opinion would give me a more positive prognosis and, although there was nothing at all lacking in my relationship with the Spanish doctor who was treating me at the time, I instinctively felt that I needed to talk to another experienced professional. There was also the issue of whether my treatment would be easier to cope with if it took place in the country of my mother-tongue. My UK-based family were quietly hoping that I would return to be close to them so that they could help in my recovery.

The second opinion agreed with the first diagnosis, a lumpectomy: 'a wide excision of the breast tumour together with a margin of normal tissue also with a lymph node assessment' would be required. The English consultant did not recommend a bi-lateral mastectomy. He felt that, as he put it: 'in the clinical context, this more radical surgery' was unlikely to give me any additional protection. Some lymph nodes may be removed in order to establish whether metastasis (the spreading of the disease) had occurred, and the type of further treatment I would receive would then be decided.

However, the UK Surgeon agreed that he would perform a bi-lateral mastectomy if that was what I wanted, although he did not feel it was necessary. The jury is still out on whether a mastectomy will offer further insurance against the cancer returning. Some of the experts I spoke to said that, with my history of fibrocystic breast disease, I was sitting on a time bomb. Other people told me that there was a slight chance that the cancer could return following a mastectomy and, therefore, this radical operation offered no further protection. I have since read that there is a one percent chance of the breast cancer returning (if there is no metastasis, of course) when you have a mastectomy. Instinctively, I felt that having a bi-lateral mastectomy was the right approach for me.

At this stage, one hopeful piece of information that I was given by the UK Consultant, following his physical examination of me, was that he didn't see a sick lady in front of him and that he was sure that my prognosis was good. This, for a time, gave us a much needed boost of confidence in my chance of surviving this dreadful disease because, up until then, I was sure that I was going to die! Although at no time did Richard express this view, I had been with him long enough to know that he was of the same mind.

I have since realised that these thoughts are born out of ignorance of the facts and the hideous way in which our society deals with the subject of cancer. I was to discover that so many people still find it difficult to mention the word, 'the Big C,' and are embarrassed when they meet you. One or two individuals found it so hard to cope that the subject was ignored altogether and I hardly ever heard from them during my treatment period. Other people are very dismissive and talk about the subject as though you were talking about the price of eggs. The impression they give is that, as statistics show that there is a higher survival rate for people with breast cancer, there is no need to worry!

On the whole, most of our family and friends coped amazingly with the news, lending an ear at any time, day or night, even if they didn't want to be reminded that we are all so vulnerable at any time to receiving such shocking news.

Following the UK meeting with the consultant, Richard and I discussed the way forward and knew that we had to make a decision relatively quickly about what type of operation I would have and where it would take place. We had provisionally booked a date for the operation the following week with the Spanish surgeon. On returning to the warm climate of Spain, away from the wet and damp of a UK November, I realised that, although we would be surrounded by family if I had the operation in the UK, it was more practical to remain at home in Spain, in my familiar surroundings. The sunshine would aid recovery and it would mean that I could sit outside or take a stroll, enjoying the fresh sea air.

Both consultants had impressed me in different ways and, although the diagnosis and prognosis were the same in both countries, I knew that the techniques used, operating procedures and the approach to convalescence would have subtle differences. This was not a problem for me as I had complete faith in the Spanish medical profession after the experience we had had when Richard had received major back surgery in 2005.

So the date was set and, listening mainly to my instincts as no one I had consulted could give me a definitive answer, I agreed to a bi-lateral mastectomy.

Chapter 4

Do or Die

FOR those of you who have experienced cancer or who know someone who has, I do not need to emphasise how this particular journey can be extremely hard at times and, for me, there were many dark, frightening moments along the way.

When I was first given my diagnosis, I felt that I was entering a tunnel and, as with most tunnels, there had to be a light at the end of it and it wasn't going to be a celestial one either! I certainly was not ready to die at fifty-three years old, especially as my first grandchild had been born six months previously. With all due respect to my God and, trust me, you really do need some sort of God to hang on to during your blackest moments, I had no intentions of letting go of my earthly existence and I continued to pray many times to Him to let me stay the course for many more years to come.

However, I am wise enough to know that any God would not send a thunderbolt to heal me. There had to be another way towards the light that I knew was at the end of the tunnel and it was up to me to make the journey to reach this goal. 'Do or die' was how I felt.

Fortunately, once the decision had been made, I did not have to wait long for the operation and, within two weeks of the biopsy result, I found myself sitting with Richard at 8.30am in the basement of a rather grand Málaga villa that has served as a private hospital for over a hundred years.

The hospital was still being run by the descendants of the original founder, Dr José Gálvez, and is located in the historic centre of Málaga City. Established in the early nineteen hundreds, the Clínica María Auxiliadora-Sanatorio del Dr Gálvez, as it was known, had pioneered a lot of medical advances brought by Dr Gálvez from Germany. In the beginning, its primary objective was to deliver successfully many babies into the world. However, it now provides many other services and the beautifully-restored building serves its purpose well, as I was soon to testify.

Within the basement was the X-ray department, pathology lab and various other clinics. With butterflies somersaulting in my tummy, whilst waiting to be called for my pre-op tests, the hustle and bustle that usually surrounds a group of Spaniards was a welcome distraction.

It is very common in Spain that, when a person is admitted into hospital, they are accompanied by members of their family, and today was no exception as there were many Spanish patients chatting away with their entourage of relatives. The family provides the carer's role that has been, to date, the traditional role of the nursing staff in UK hospitals. The Spanish nursing staff tend to take a more proactive role in administering any medical care required. I wondered if these particular Spanish patients thought Richard and I were a lonely pair sitting there without any relations to keep us company!

Feeling thirsty and sick with hunger and fear - I was not allowed any breakfast as the operation had been scheduled for 11.00 that morning - I suddenly noticed, walking towards us, our very dear Spanish friend, Paulino, with a rather large grin on his face. He greeted us warmly and we made some joke about how great it was to see that our Spanish family had arrived.

Paulino was a headmaster at a Primary School in a village not far from where we lived and had school business to attend to in Málaga. He had decided to make a detour to the hospital in order to ensure that we were both coping with the situation. This was a welcome relief, especially for Richard, as they could have coffee together, he could chat to Paulino, if necessary, about his concerns and, as Paulino always made us laugh, they could share a few jokes, too.

I am not sure whether it was at this point that an ongoing joke emerged, that would humorously plague my life over the coming months, about my eventual need for reconstruction surgery. I had been offered the opportunity for the reconstruction of my breasts at the same time as the double mastectomy but had declined as I felt that I had enough to cope with and, never being particularly vain, I was not really interested in the subject at that stage. My prime objective was to become a positive statistic: one of the millions of breast cancer victims who had survived. Therefore, reconstruction was really the last thing on my mind.

However, this did not stop the jokes that would come fast and furious and, at this point in the proceedings, I didn't mind. In fact, I often encouraged the humour that this subject inspired. I was fast realising that, within this great black tunnel that I had entered, there were some welcome respites and humour was one of them.

Although, within our relationship, Richard is probably the more quick-witted, as is our son, I have always recognised the need to embrace constructive humour (I am not a great lover of mocking others just for the sake of it). There are many opportunities for irony, situational and mild black humour, which sometimes relieve the stress and tension of everyday tragedies and there have been countless occasions that I have found humour a welcome relief from the blackness of a situation.

Laughter is a great tonic and we should have regular doses of it. I often reflect with fondness and a chuckle at the comically strange situations that occurred during John's funeral all those years ago - like the time my mother visited the Chapel of Rest with us and, seeing John's body lying there, proceeded to touch him. Her hands travelled down to his legs and suddenly she exclaimed in her broad South Wales accent; 'Where's his legs? He's got no legs!' I can remember peering over the coffin, trying to stifle my giggles, and tried to reassure her that in fact he still had two legs. Goodness knows where she thought they had gone as he had not lost them in the accident. The body does shrink following death, however!

Another occasion where I did, in fact, burst into hysterical laughter was during the transportation of John's ashes in the oak cask from the funeral parlour to our home. I collected them one stormy day, accompanied by my daughter, sister-in-law and my mother. Standing by the car, I was suddenly tickled by the need to make the decision as to where to put the casket whilst travelling home. It wasn't fair to ask my passengers to balance the box on their knees and I was certainly not happy about leaving the casket in the boot of the car. Eventually, it was settled that my sister-law would hold him. As I climbed into the car, I quipped; "I wasn't happy about letting my son roll around in the boot all the way home". This was tragic but funny, also. John would have laughed as he shared the same black sense of humour as his father and brother.

At times, my head felt as though it would explode with all of the fears, thoughts and concerns that were starting to mount. When these panic attacks first commenced, they would be accompanied with an overwhelming sense of gratitude for Richard. My husband was proving to be not only my great comforter when these horrendous uncertainties emerged but he showered me with even more affection than usual. His demonstrative actions certainly improved my self-esteem and I enveloped myself in this security blanket when everything became too much to cope with.

When we talk about those times, Richard insists that I was so strong and positive about our predicament that it helped him - maybe I was. All I felt at the time was that his rock solid support and love gave me the strength I needed to make the journey that was ahead of me. Overall, the cancer journey was travelled together with our family in tow. They were with us every step of the way, especially our children. However, there were moments when I felt very alone and lost, unsure as to whether I was making the right decisions, such as the time when I was admitted into theatre for the mastectomy. Panic set in as I lay down on the operating table and I just felt like jumping up and running away.

During those moments of panic, which often came at night, I turned to prayer. Throughout my life I had always prayed to God - not only in times of crisis but also when something productive and rewarding had happened to me or if I needed guidance with a particular problem. I had always found great solace within this spiritual prayer, which usually took place in my head. However, I will admit that, from the time Oliver died, my faith had waned somewhat and the innate spirituality that intuitively accompanied me on my journey through life was dimming. I could not seem to justify the reason Oliver had died and losing my enthusiasm for my spiritual values contributed greatly to the demise of the positive traits of my once energetic personality.

On reflection, for a long time, I had been operating like a robot and just going through the motions of living. I remember our daughter asking me, in the September before the diagnosis, if I was depressed. I denied it, of course, as I didn't feel depressed, just tired. Being the sensitive, intuitive woman she is, she knew something was wrong before I did!

Growing up and travelling into the journey of adulthood, I had always tried to ensure that I maintained a compassionate social conscience, helping others where necessary. It did not matter whether their need was emotional or physical, I tried to be there for my family and friends, as I felt instinctively that this was the right way to behave as my interpretation of God had always been there for me. When I have felt weak, a prayer would help me feel strong and, if I was angry or tormented, talking to Him helped to calm me down.

I always feel that I am watched over and, when there is a crisis or if I need to be shown a different approach and behave more humbly in life, the correct way inevitably comes to mind. However, if I become too overconfident or selfish, which happens to us all from time to time, like any good father, He presents circumstances to show me that you should never become too self-assured.

What proof, you may ask, do I have that it is my God that advises me and not just my conscience. Have you ever experienced a situation where you are feeling pretty awful about something or you are very worried about a particular situation and, suddenly, out of nowhere appears a solution? Many times, I have become too sure, too stubborn or too self-satisfied that all is well in my life. Circumstances, without warning, change rapidly or a new opportunity presents itself and I find myself thinking that I wasn't so in control as I had thought. This is not always coincidence, I feel, as it happens too frequently.

When I reflect on the events leading up to that awful night in November, 1990, when John died, several factors show that during this time I was feeling very complacent and over-confident about certain areas of my life.

Richard and I had had just come through a difficult period in our marriage. He had not been totally convinced by my decision to risk starting a business and, although he had been a great support and had eventually given up his teaching job to join me in the business, he needed convincing that, in the long term, the business would grow and be successful. However, we seemed to have passed through this period and we were starting to benefit from the improved lifestyle, taking nice family holidays to places like Florida or weekend breaks away together, when time permitted. The children were doing well at school and, looking back, I can now see how a comfortable blanket of complacency had settled over our family life.

I remember feeling quite self-satisfied and very confident that the future would continue to go well for the business and for my family.

The learning experience I have taken from that period when John died was to believe that no matter how full your cup is at any moment in your life, do not lose your humility, continue to feel grateful for what you have; thank God that life is good and never become too self-assured about family and friends. Always be aware of what a wonderful world is around you. Just enjoy the moment! We should never worry about the future as God (if you believe in Him) or fate will take care of that.

How many times have I wished I could abide by the following words:

"God, grant me the serenity
to accept the things I cannot change,
the courage to change the things I can,
and the wisdom to know the difference."

CHAPTER 5

A SPANISH MEDICAL EXPERIENCE

COMING round in the recovery room, following the operation, was a strange experience. The last thing I had remembered before the operation, following the anxious walk into the operating theatre and climbing on to the operating table (I had not received a pre-med before my general anaesthetic), was asking God, quietly within myself, for strength to cope with the fear of what lay ahead. Somewhere in the background, the doctor who was responsible for placing the oxygen mask over my face was joking with me about my Spanish not being very fluent considering that I had been living in Spain for eight years.

As I began to wake up, two and half hours later, my eyes took a while to focus again and I was conscious that I was 'rabbiting' on in Spanish to the two nurses attending me. They were busy checking my blood pressure, the drips and drains. I seemed to be trying to prove that I could, in fact, speak some Spanish after all as I took them through a detailed description of my family. They politely ignored me and allowed me to drone on in my anaesthetic-drunken state. Suddenly my diatribe ceased as I couldn't remember the Spanish word for grandson, and Richard arrived.

A big smile from him gave me the reassurance I needed, that I had survived this stage of my journey. I tried to converse with him but my teeth would not stop chattering from either the cold or the shock of the operation and so he just held my hand.

It was not long before I was wheeled to a very comfortable private room with a sleep sofa for Richard, who would be staying with me. I became conscious of two strange tubes, one protruding from my left side and one from my right side, as I was lifted from the theatre trolley on to my bed. Wincing with pain, it was becoming very apparent that, if I wanted to keep discomfort to a minimum, I needed to treat them with due consideration.

Once settled in bed, I realised that I would not be going too far for a while. Although I was receiving painkillers intravenously and the whole of my chest area felt numb, I could not move to the left or right for obvious reasons. The pain was too dreadful. I later discovered that I had been cut from under one armpit, right across my chest, to the other armpit.

It was late afternoon when our Spanish 'family' returned to offer support and help with my bed care. Paulino's wife, Luisa, kindly offered me small sips of water and generally fussed over me in a bid to make sure I was as comfortable as possible.

Our daughter had expressed a desire to support her father while I was in hospital. However, she had a baby to consider and hospital is not the most congenial of environments for a small child, despite the fact that the Spanish welcome little children with open arms. As I would only be in hospital for a maximum of a week, I thought it would better if she delayed her visit until I was discharged and she could also then help her father to care for me at home.

Our son was coming over to Spain from the Middle East, where he was currently working, for Christmas and he managed to extend his leave to three weeks, to include the holiday period and, more importantly, to be involved in our impending move at the beginning of December into a new apartment.

Our children were towers of strength, giving sound advice despite being involved in such a difficult situation and they were always available to listen if I needed to express my concerns and worries. It could not have been easy to watch their mother become so debilitated, lose her normal abundant levels of energy and be involved in reversing parent-child roles. I would often lie awake at night feeling sick with worry that they were having difficulty coping with the situation. I knew that I had to try to quell these moments of worry as they would certainly not aid my recovery. It was a very good learning opportunity for me to experience the letting go of my children, something I have found difficult to do at times, realising that they are adults and need to be able to cope with whatever life throws at them.

Each child is so different, but all three of ours inherited their father's sensitive and intuitive nature so I knew that, deep down, they would probably have moments of torment about whether their mother would survive this dreadful disease.

Survive I would, this much I had promised myself as I lay awake the whole of the first night after my operation. I felt pretty uncomfortable from the surgery but the worst aspect of that night was an overpowering sensation of drowning: that my wonderful life was slipping away. The intense fear of dying had hit me with full force and I have never been so scared in my life. John was constantly in my thoughts since Richard and I had both realised that my diagnosis date had been seventeen years exactly to the day that he had died and my operation took place on the seventeenth anniversary of his funeral.

I hung on to my life force as I tried to put these agonising thoughts out of my head. I found myself praying so hard for strength to get me through what lay ahead in the coming months. I gave thanks for everything I had and asked that I would recover and be able to grow old with my darling husband, continue to be part of our children's lives and watch our grandchildren grow up. I wasn't asking for much! All night I was conscious there was someone other than Richard with me in the room. I am absolutely convinced that Lucas, the dear, elderly Greek friend who had died in September, was holding my crossed hands as they lay on my stomach.

During this time I felt comforted by the fact that my inner strength and belief were returning and that the power of prayer was re-entering my life. In the previous weeks, leading up to the operation, I had received numerous kind messages of support and often there would be references to prayers held for me and advice on how to ask my angels for help. The gifts of cards, spiritual artefacts and flowers

I had received all helped to encourage me to return to the spiritual path that I had virtually abandoned when Oliver had died two years previously.

Never before had I needed my God as much as at that moment in my life and I was certainly not going to let my children down by not being around to help them when they needed me. However, what unfolded during the following days in hospital demonstrated to me that a full recovery would be a long road to travel and that this was just the beginning.

Inspired by my new-found strength of will, which promised to assist me during my journey through cancer and the desire not to use the bed pan, I was determined to get out of bed on the morning after the operation. As soon as the nurse arrived to give me a bed bath, on the second day, I asked her if I would be allowed to get out of bed that morning. She agreed and promised to return. True to her word, a short while later she came and helped me out of bed. Swinging my drains gently to each side, Richard took one arm and the nurse took the other and the aim was to walk me towards the armchair a few feet away from the bed.

All was going well until I sat down and suddenly I felt every ounce of strength and energy leave my body and I was conscious of slumping forward. A voice in my head repeatedly reinforced the need for me to keep upright and to hang on because I hadn't seen my children. All three of them were with me, larger than life, and all I can say is that a huge wave of instinctive love for my children engulfed me and blocked my life-force from draining away.

As I felt my eyes roll back in my head and I had difficulty

in breathing, my thoughts were that I must not die or even pass out. The nurse ran out of the room and returned seconds later with a male colleague who proceeded to insert something into my mouth. Instantly I felt my breathing improve and, although very nauseous, I was relieved that the floating sensation was leaving me.

They helped me back to bed and I realised that, in my impatience to kick-start my road to recovery, it was not such a good idea to be rushing out of bed so soon after the operation. But then, patience has never been a virtue of mine and, over the coming months, situations would present themselves, which would test me time and time again - all part of the character changes I would endure, some of which I welcomed and others which would prove to be a real struggle to accept.

As the days passed in hospital, slowly, with Richard's help, I managed to become more mobile, avoiding whenever possible looking at the disfigurement that I knew was there as a result of having no boobs! Initially, I was also a little coy with Richard; although at no time did he ever make me feel self-conscious about my appearance. However, very soon this coyness would melt away as I realised how much I depended on him for help to shower and get dressed.

Once the drains were removed from my sides, I found getting around and sleeping a lot more comfortable. On the second day, the surgeon arrived and, as I was getting out of bed for him to examine me, he proceeded to explain that the operation had gone very well and that he would have the complete results of further tests that they had needed to carry out in about a week. He kindly stated that he would ensure I would still be around in ten years time!

Although I knew full well that this statement was probably tongue in cheek, I was overwhelmed with gratitude and started to cry. He embraced me with the usual Spanish style kiss on each cheek, gave me a hug and then examined me, proudly explaining how well everything was healing.

What a task he had trying to save women like me from succumbing to this dreadful disease. I was still at the stage in my journey where fear kept raising its ugly head and I hung on to any morsel of information that gave me some hope that I really would still be around in ten years. He visited me every day and I was so impressed that he attended to the dressing of the wounds himself, treating my body like a work of art, not even allowing the nurse who attended a chance to show off her nursing skills.

The decision to give myself over to this amazing surgeon had been proved to be the right one. At this stage, I realised that, once you have made the choice about the type of treatment and operation that you are going to undergo, it is so important to have faith and complete trust in your surgeon's abilities. Your life really is in their hands but that does not mean to say that you don't question everything that is going on at the time. A good surgeon should encourage your inquisitiveness.

Although still weak, by the fourth day, I was ready to go home. Sleeping in hospital is always difficult and we were delighted when the doctor discharged me. Getting dressed to go home was difficult as I still could not move my arms above my waist and I was becoming very aware of how much you use your chest muscles when you walk.

Losing your breasts also deprives you of the warmth that they provide at the front of your chest and rib-cage and, when I stepped outside the hospital, that November morning, the cold Spanish Levante wind suddenly hit me. Trying to get into the car proved difficult, too, and it was impossible to shut the door without a searing pain rushing through my whole body. Physical adjustments for manoeuvring my body needed to be made, and quickly, if I was going to survive without painkillers. On leaving hospital, I had not been offered any medication to take home and I was determined to find an alternative way of coping with the pain. I was not keen to bombard my system with any more drugs, especially as it was possible that I would have to undergo Chemotherapy.

The forty-five kilometre journey home proved difficult as every time Richard's foot hit the brake the jarring would move the upper part of my body. By folding my arms gently across my chest I managed to keep this area as still as possible.

As is often the case when you are in hospital, you acquire a false sense of wellness, and this occasion proved no different. I felt that I had coped quite well with the pain as I lay in my hospital bed, only moving to use the bathroom or getting up to have meals. Once the drips had been removed, I was not aware that I was given any further pain killers and only one night did I require a sleeping pill and that was due to the noise of the hospital. Once we had arrived home at the apartment (we were renting until our new one was completed), the pain management proved to be a different story.

CHAPTER 6

HOME SWEET HOME

THE first few days settling back into Civvy Street are a little blurred and seem to have been a constant battle to carry out all bodily functions in the slowest and most pain-free way possible. Sleeping was extremely difficult as to lie down was shear agony and I could only really get comfortable if my side was propped up by pillows. Richard tried to emulate the layout of the hospital pillows which allowed my arms to be elevated at right angles when I was in bed. To get up involved my sitting bolt upright, using my stomach muscles to thrust my body forward, all the time being careful to ensure I was taking pressure or strain off my chest muscles or what I felt was left of them.

Naturally, I was keen to be as independent as I could because I felt that this would be good psychologically both for me and for my loved ones if it looked as though I was returning to my normal role as wife, mother and grandmother. After all, although physical changes had occurred on the outside of my body, I was still the same person inside. This proved to be a big mistake and, within a few days, several situations occurred to remind me of exactly what condition I was in both mentally and physically.

Although I managed to carry out my daily shower independently, I was still avoiding eye contact with any mirrors. It was important that Richard was available to run the shower as it was impossible to reach up to the controls and also for him to help me in and out of the shower. Dressing the lower half of my body proved easier than the top half for obvious reasons and, often, I would keep my pyjamas and dressing gown on for most of the day. Without my competent carer and life partner, I often thought where would I be?

Our family had wanted to come over immediately to support Richard and to help where they could. However, there are times when you need to be firm and practical about help and visitation for their sake as well as your own. My siblings were working full-time and their offers of help were much appreciated. However, it was not sensible to involve them at this stage and I knew that I would be seeing my mother and elder sister at Christmas so I persuaded them to stay put in the UK as I was in very capable hands. Fortunately my best friend and Oliver's mother, Paula, also offered to help with the move and flew over from France. She proved to be an invaluable asset during the first few days of my recovery period.

Our wonderful Spanish, Norwegian and English friends that lived on the Costa del Sol rallied round and carried out practical tasks such as supplying us with abundant amounts of homemade soup and meals on wheels!

After a few difficult days and feeling very desperate that the pain and discomfort were not easing, I noticed a leaflet that I had left on the coffee table which detailed a local homeopathic therapist.

Before entering hospital I had promised myself that, once the operation was over, I would commence, in earnest, my research into what could be done to free myself of the cancer and to ensure it did not return by using complementary therapies alongside the orthodox approach. I had always been an avid enthusiast of natural approaches to keeping healthy and fit and, as far as I was concerned, this life situation would prove no different. My initial question was where was my starting point? I soon discovered that the first step was in pain management and making contact with the homeopathic therapist was perhaps what I was looking for.

Since my diagnosis, I had been given several articles and books on the subject of cancer from well-meaning family and friends. Although information is extremely useful, when you are frightened and confused it can cause you to become more worried as you assimilate various sometimes-contradictory points. One such point was haunting me and I raised this, when, within the first week, I made a trip to my GP for a check up. Fortunately my gynaecologist was at the clinic that day and I was able to ask her a few questions about the niggling concerns I had such as what were the chances of the cancer returning to my chest area now that I no longer had breasts?

Both professionals informed me that there was a slim possibility and that, because of my history of benign breast disease, if I had not had both breasts removed, I would have been sitting on a time bomb!

An examination reassured me that the healing was making good progress and I didn't raise the subject of taking any medication for the pain as I knew that pain-killers were only a short-term remedy. I knew, also, that it was very important not to bombard my liver with too many drugs as it was likely to have enough to deal with when or if I was prescribed chemotherapy. Keeping the liver as clean as possible was to become a high priority in my quest for complementary therapy.

An appointment was made to see the complementary therapist, whom I shall call Joan. I wasn't sure what to expect when she arrived for her first consultation with me and I was surprised to discover that the hour and half appointment was conducted mainly as an interview with questioning regarding not only my health record but my life's experiences. This proved somewhat surprising as my original request had simply been to provide me with a natural painkiller.

Joan explained that homeopathic treatment was not just about providing a cure but that it was more important to treat the patient holistically through understanding what was the likely cause and effect of the ailment. This is carried out through the analysis of the individual's mental and physical condition, taking into consideration any weaknesses or ailments that they may have encountered. Once the analysis was complete, the information was fed into a comprehensive database which would search for suggested treatments.

My first meeting proved to be fruitful in several ways. First and foremost, it certainly was beneficial to have someone from outside my family, who didn't know me, to talk about my situation and experiences to date. As you will appreciate, there is only so much talking you can do with your kith and kin without feeling the need to protect them from too much worry.

The therapist was very probing in her style of approach, more like a counsellor, and she soon opened up several areas of my life which I thought were tucked safely away. Very simplistically, on a mental level, it was identified that fear was an issue that I had difficulty in resolving and this would often manifest itself in unreasonable anxieties about my children and family. It was evident that the cause of some of this fear could be traced back to my childhood and, instead of confronting those fears, I had buried them. As is often the case with unresolved mind issues, they may remain dormant for some time and may come to the fore, appearing at a later stage in one's life.

Another issue that began to occur to me when I was being questioned by the therapist was my inability to control my drive to achieve as much as I can in a day and in my life, and how little time, since we gave up our company, Richard and I spent relaxing. Some people, when they retire, have difficulty occupying their days. However, that never proved to be a problem for us as I drove us on to achieve as much as we physically could in a day. Weekends didn't exist in Spain as we would be busy from Monday morning to Sunday night. When we visited the children in the UK, it would be no different as we always wanted to help them as much as we could.

Holiday times sometimes proved more restful but only if we checked into a hotel. Even then, I would insist that we visited all the sights and museums, and underwent some kind of physical exercise every day. If I failed to be satisfied with what I had achieved, I would feel a sense of failure and that I had let myself and others down. I would often say that I could not be doing with sitting around all day, not achieving! Little did I realise that it is actually good for you to daydream a little, take time out to just be. I am certainly learning to do that now and my grandson, Louis-John, has had a helping hand in this change in my life

The beating myself up model that I had discovered while undergoing this therapy and which had become an integral part of my character, was not necessarily the therapist's desired outcome from the initial interview, and subsequent meetings and the releasing from me of a lot of emotion was certainly not on her agenda either. As the flood gates opened on more than one occasion, it certainly made me feel better, gave me food for thought and the determination to sort out the reasons why I was on this particular journey.

The impression I got was that Joan needed a factual record of my medical history and any relevant examples of stressful situations that I had so far encountered in my life. Giving as much information as I could remember, she went away to carry out the analysis, leaving behind some very small white pills in two envelopes, one marked belladonna and the other arnica. I was told that I could take the arnica as and when I felt the need as this would help with the healing inside, and any bruising. The belladonna tablets were to be taken one in the morning and one at night and, only if the burning pain became really unbearable, should I increase the dosage.

These little white pills proved a great help in the management of the pain during the healing process and, whenever I forgot to take one or if I decided to cut them back, the discomfort would return within a short while.

A week after the first meeting with the homoeopathist, she telephoned me to say that she had found a possible solution to part of my problem. At this stage, I only saw my cancer as the problem and solving this particular problem was in the hands of the doctors. I felt that, by introducing me to the little white pills, she had helped me enormously so I was curious to discover what further help she was offering.

In describing my medical history and any ailments that had plagued me, I had given Joan such details as chronic PMT (pre-menstrual tension), painful periods, three difficult child-births, benign breast disease from my mid-twenties, uterine fibroids, a hysterectomy (including the removal of my ovaries), difficulty in sleeping, blood sugar imbalance (if I didn't eat every two to three hours I would be like a demented animal), and, finally, breast cancer!

She had explained that it had taken quite a while to identify a solution from feeding the above medical details into the database. However, eventually she had discovered a common thread running through all of the information. They all linked to an imbalance in iodine and she was going to prescribe a substance called Iodium. Iodium, also known as iodine, is a popular homeopathic mineral choice for many homeopaths who are presented with people facing glandular problems. Since glands affect many other aspects of bodily functions, the use of iodium to get to the root of many health problems is extremely common.

The substance arrived with a pipette and I was instructed to put five drops in half a tumbler of water in the morning and make up a fresh amount at night. After taking a teaspoon of the mixture, I was to throw the rest away. The most bizarre action I had to carry out was as follows: before I put the drops into the half glass of water, I had to tap the bottle ten to fifteen times and this gentle banging of the bottle should be increased if I needed to increase the number of drops. The percussion seemed to allow the highly diluted iodium to change its constitution and it was important that the substance was mixed thoroughly before I ingested it.

I was advised to monitor the way I was feeling and keep the therapist informed of any changes that I experienced. Immediately, my blood sugar imbalance improved and I started to sleep better. I would have wobbly days where my blood sugar felt out of balance and I knew that I would have to watch what, and how frequently, I ate. In previous years, I had undergone tests for diabetes and there was no evidence to suggest that I was a diabetic. Perhaps, I thought, I was suffering from hyperglycaemia. Therefore, I knew my diet was crucial in controlling how I felt.

If my symptoms continued to worsen, I was told that I should increase the number of drops and percussions. I eventually increased the number of drops to twenty, morning and night. I can certainly say that the symptoms that had bothered me over the last few years such as the blood-sugar problem and waking up constantly at night did improve during this period, although they didn't go away entirely. That may have been due to other physiological changes that were happening at the time.

Joan felt that I may have to continue using the iodium for the rest of my life. However, I continued to use it for seven months and I still have a supply if, at any time, my condition deteriorates.

The experience of this type of complementary therapy proved to be my introduction to the many naturopathic approaches that exist to treat a whole host of diseases and this led me on to discover that there are hundreds of treatment methods and suggested cures for cancer. None of those I came across had been scientifically proven to be one hundred per cent successful but many individuals had been cured or had gone into remission, convinced that the particular remedy they had discovered had helped them.

During the next few months I had some very useful follow-up meetings and at one such meeting Joan introduced me to a very interesting book and DVD entitled "The Secret" by Rhonda Byrne (ISBN 9781847370297, Published by Simon and Schuster Ltd).

Simplistically, "The Secret" outlines the philosophy that we have the power to change our life dramatically through believing in constructive thoughts and actions, and utilising the positive energy that is emanating from the universe, or God, depending on what your convictions are. We can achieve anything we desire through the law of attraction by consciously thinking about, involving ourselves in and working towards the chosen goal.

The book proved to be an inspiration and helped me at this point in my journey through cancer. It showed me once again, how in life, opportunities and objects present themselves to teach you how to become stronger and more positive. I felt that I was at last returning to a more spiritual path

Inspired by the motivational techniques I found in this book I knew that I would reach my chosen goal, which was to rid myself of cancer. The inspirational contents of the DVD moved me to encourage everyone I came in contact with to watch it! Very few people could refuse my persuasive suggestion and I am sure many watched the contents just to pacify me!

The DVD included several interviews with successful individuals, as well as ordinary people, who gave examples of how using The Secret had worked for them.

One particular lady's experience interested me. She had discovered a cancerous lump in her breast and had refused treatment. Throughout the first three months, following her diagnosis, she spent a lot of her time surrounding herself with positive people, with abundant amounts of laughter by watching humorous films and had tried to avoid contact with anyone negative or miserable. When she returned for her check up, the doctors were astounded that the cancer had disappeared. These were just the stories that I wanted to hear as I continued my journey through cancer.

CHAPTER 7

YOU ARE WHAT YOU EAT

ON my return from hospital, my short-term objectives were to search for a method and approach for managing the day-to-day pain and to try to organise my daily routine. Once these objectives were under control, the medium to longer-term ones, I was sure, would become evident.

The main daily focus became a quest to discover a recovery strategy to restore myself as quickly as possible to total health. Tackling the disease by using the orthodox approach alongside a complementary therapy, if I could find one, seemed the most sensible course of action. Using our very best research skills, Richard and I ferociously attacked the Internet. We read and devoured incredible amounts of information, becoming increasingly confused as to where the complementary health protocol I was going to adopt should commence.

The first discovery we made was a book, "Cancer-Free, Your Guide to Gentle, Non-Toxic Healing" by Bill Henderson, from the website,

www.beating-cancer-gently.com.

Bill Henderson, an American from Florida, speaks from

experience. He lost his wife to cancer after she battled with the disease for four years and has spent many years, following her death, studying, researching, attending seminars and lectures and listening to individuals' experiences and examples of complementary approaches to the subject of healing cancer through self-help. In his quest to help others, he spends every day communicating by e-mail and telephone with cancer patients and he claims: 'I am not a doctor. I am just a reporter. However, with the information I have gathered, I have been able to help hundreds of people all over the world become cancer-free.'

I quickly downloaded the e-book while Richard excitedly bombarded me with pages and pages of printouts all boasting recommended cures. These included details of herbal concoctions, vitamin supplements, tinctures, teas and homeopathic substances fighting cancer by increasing cellular oxygen levels, killing cancer cells with cellulite. The list was endless.

While I focused on the detail of what the products professed to do and tried to analyse the appropriate way forward, Richard revealed many web-sites from experts in the field of breast cancer and filtered through them as best he could. It wasn't mentally or physically possible to take everything on board, in the time I felt I had available, and we both became very apt at skimming the Internet, sifting out the quackery and what we deemed to be poor quality products for sale.

Bill Henderson's e-book quickly became a lifeline and, although there are seven comprehensive chapters to read, packed with useful information, as I was in a hurry to commence my protocol immediately, I skimmed the first four chapters and headed for chapter five: 'Cancer Self-

Treatments That I Recommend.' I was especially interested in the sub-section on immune-building.

Nutrition and understanding the correlation between what you eat and health has always been of interest to me. Indeed, some family members would say that this is an obsession. I like to think that it is more of a hobby and, over the years, I have collected many books on diet, cooking and health, as our bulging bookcase proves. Therefore, when I started to read this newly discovered book, I wasn't surprised to hear a strong message coming out of the pages: 'YOU ARE WHAT YOU EAT'.

Another subject, which was emphasised as being extremely important and which kept coming up time and time again in all the other literature we read, was the importance of a strong immune-system when trying to cure cancer. Obviously a body with a strong defence system is needed to avoid contracting cancer in the first place or any other disease for that matter and it becomes even more vital when you are struck down with a disease.

As I absorbed the reading matter that I had started to accumulate, I was delighted to re-discover this vital key to restoring my health and that it was totally in my hands. To many, it may seem as though I am stating the obvious and, as is often the case in life, the simplest of solutions can be overlooked, and especially when you feel that time is running out.

The first stage in devising my strategy for a natural approach to ridding myself of the cancer completely had got to be in restoring and re-building my immune-system. The question was how to do this quickly. Diet had to be a factor in the equation and detailed in our research were numerous examples of products purporting to assist in the rebuilding of the immune-system.

How was I to choose the products that would be the most effective? That was the next question and, because I was still experiencing feelings of total panic, I became very confused and the nagging belief that I needed to make a decision fast would not go away. This is when I turned to the concise but comprehensive information in Bill Henderson's book.

Coincidentally, I had received a telephone call from Joan to tell me she had discovered what looked like a very good book on curing cancer naturally, written by a certain Bill Henderson! We both agreed that he seemed very experienced and that his motives for writing the book were genuine. This telephone call spurred me on to review, once again, the contents of chapter five of Bill's book and to concentrate my efforts in one area for the time being.

Details of some eight proven products to help in restoring the immune-system were outlined in detail in chapter five. Fortunately, it did not prove difficult to make the decision which of the eight options I would use because there was a recommendation that three of the eight were probably the most effective.

I was anxious to get started as soon as possible and, because these products were being ordered from the USA, I knew that there was no time to waste. Another reason I was determined to move so quickly was the thought of having Chemotherapy – presenting an even more pressing need for building up my natural defence system.

Although I was still a few days away from receiving the results of the tests carried out during my operation, I was aware of the need to prepare my body in case it had to deal with the onslaught of such debilitating drugs. As you will probably have guessed, I had also started to research into the side effects and content of the drugs used by the medical profession to combat cancer, and I didn't like what I was reading! What I was deducing from the research was that the chemotherapy can have significantly negative effects on the white and red cells of the blood, the liver and the kidneys. Therefore, simplistically, if the white cells contribute to the body's immune system, I knew that it was going to be doubly important that my immune-system was strong from the outset.

Diet was also now becoming more of a priority as I realised that my liver and kidneys would need all the help they could receive to clean and strengthen them from the onslaught of the chemicals.

I noticed that, alongside the constant state of panic I was feeling at this time, another emotion was emerging - a growing sense of excitement as I felt a sense of "Eureka!" - I was finding an answer to one of the questions that had been plaguing me: What could I do to help myself? At this stage in my recovery, I realised that, because I was a novice at understanding complementary therapy, it would be very difficult to be fully committed to all of the recommendations I was discovering in Bill Henderson's e-book. Therefore, I decided, rather quickly, that the starting point for me had to be to feed my body with at least three products that I had identified and chosen from the list of eight in the e-book and to finalise the correct diet that would boost my defence mechanisms naturally. It sounded easy!

Now all I had to do was to convince Richard and our daughter, Paula, who was currently visiting, that it was important to establish a routine whereby the health protocol and recovery plan could be put into place. I knew that I needed to get them both on board if this was going to be a success.

CHAPTER 8

FALLING APART

IN the early days, Richard and Paula were my main carers and were responsible for organising meals, both on time as well as the right content of the meal - a quick ham sandwich was definitely not on the menu. It was all I could do to dress myself and ensure that I was taking all of the vitamin supplements as outlined in my new complementary protocol. They were numerous and, at one stage, I was swallowing over forty supplements a day.

Maybe I wasn't very clear about how to communicate the importance and the urgency of my new regime. Cooking had never been Richard's forte. He had always left it to me, saying that I was far better at pulling together quickly an appetising and healthy meal. He always found eating a chore, though he had always been happy to assist me with meal preparation. Therefore, initially, meal times were anything but on time and it was difficult for Paula to help Richard as she had brought along her new-born baby and his demands at mealtimes, quiet rightly, certainly outweighed mine.

It was even more important that I received my low-glycemic meals on time and that I ate regularly as I had decided to become practically a vegan, learning very quickly from other reliable sources that dairy and red meat were no-nos.

A lack of animal-based protein intake began to indicate to me that my overall blood-sugar was affected and, within two hours of eating, I was becoming light-headed and needed an input of calories immediately.

One day, everything seemed to come to a head. This was not surprising, considering the stress we had all been under. At the time, I was busy trying to write out the protocol of complementary medications and organise some sort of regime to follow so that I didn't forget what I should be taking. The simple task of writing was taking a considerable amount of time and proving quite painful, as any activity which disturbed my scarred chest cut through me like a knife. Richard was busy with domestic chores and lunchtime was fast approaching. Paula was feeding Louis-John so I attempted to prepare a lunch of salad. This was proving extremely difficult as I was still unable to raise my arms very high and chopping was impossible. I was also becoming increasingly bad-tempered as my blood sugar plummeted. My nerves had become rather frayed and I started to cry out of shear frustration and weakness. Richard tried to help as best he could.

Through emotional outbursts of sobbing, I tried to communicate, ineffectively, the importance of regular mealtimes and how I felt that my newly-established protocol was not being taking seriously.

With everyone's emotions getting the better of them, accusations flying around the room and self-defence mechanisms moving into place, a full scale row broke out between Richard and me, and Paula took the role of referee between her parents.

Slumping into a chair, head in hands, feeling completed exhausted, I realised that poor Richard was confused as to how he was failing me in his role as carer. I sensed that he was a little sceptical as to how I would achieve success in my quest to heal myself and was, perhaps, concerned that I was thinking about abandoning using the orthodox approach in favour of natural therapies. Well, at that stage, I wasn't entirely sure where my journey was going and how it would end. Instinctively, I just knew that doing something practical was more positive than sitting around feeling sorry for myself.

Self-pity is a behaviour I had always tried to avoid as I believe it to be pointless and destructive. If I came across a friend or family member who would demonstrate this trait, I would always try to lend a shoulder to cry on but I never felt that I needed one - until now.

In the coming months, I would come to realise the importance of occasionally allowing the indulgence of feeling sorry for myself and of acknowledging that my life had taken a difficult path. Denial or too much self-pity are not healthy and, from my experience, do not lead to a contented approach to life and relationships.

At this stage in my journey, self-piteous I was not. I was, however, both terrified and self-indulgent. It appeared that the type of help I was requesting from my two carers was not being understood very well and I needed to re-emphasise why it was necessary to heed my requests and ensure that we worked together to achieve the goal of establishing a routine for my complementary protocol. Through making my needs a priority at this stage, there was every possibility I would heal and regain my independence from my carers more rapidly, thus allowing everyone to benefit.

This sounds as though I was attacking my problem very

coldly and not giving my family the room they needed to be confused, scared and devastated. This wasn't the case and, amidst the tears, accusations and tantrums that are often displayed when a married couple argue, we tried to reach an understanding. I also realised what a huge task I was asking Richard to support me in and explained how desperate I felt.

There really was no alternative but to move forward. What else could I do, and I needed his help. Support he did and Paula's mediating actions helped calm the situation and she was able to put succinctly to us both that arguing was not helping my recovery and any further confusions and differences should be put aside. The whole incident left us all drained and exhausted and a similar blow out occurred over Christmas as, once again, I felt that my recovery regime was being side tracked and I was not keeping to the routine required to achieve my goals.

On reflection, both unfortunate rows proved to be as a result of a married couple coping with managing the changes that were happening in their lives. Each partner will have different approaches to dealing with the changes that inevitably occur when one of you has cancer. Coming to terms with the issues that an individual expresses at various times should be dealt with at their own pace.

Most of the time, Richard and I found the synergy that was needed to work together at keeping my protocol on track and I cannot fault the care and understanding that he gave me. Once he realised how proactive I needed to be on the road to my full recovery, he never failed to support me - even when that meant spending vast amounts of money on strange substances which I hoped would help me in my journey through cancer.

The profound effect that the shock of seeing his loved

one, who normally was so full of energy and life, in such a sorry state at times must have proved unbearable and, privately, there were many moments where we shed tears together and offered one another love and empathy. The trauma of everything that had happened had left us exhausted and our nerves shattered as we tried to manage the change that had been thrust upon us.

Some big adjustments were made in our relationship. Some of those were conscious and others more instinctive and unconscious. I could sense Richard's vulnerability as we attempted to redefine our roles. He took on more of the decision-making, initially some of the domestic chores, and took over more of the day-to-day organisation of our life which had primarily been my responsibility.

I helped where I could, although the soreness of the scarring would continue for some time and there were days when I would find myself depressed especially when simple tasks, such as walking on the beach, proved impossible unless I supported my arms by folding them across my chest - a strange position to hold oneself in when trying to carry out a daily exercise ritual!

Slowly, the changes were made and, together, we reached an understanding of what strategy needed to be in place to ensure that we were able to make this journey through cancer together.

During this time, and every day since, I have never taken for granted how fortunate I was not to have to work during this period and how I was able to have time to devote to my healing programme. I know that there are thousands of women who are not as fortunate as me in having the support of a devoted family and the time away from work to recover from cancer quickly and effectively; nor do they have the benefit of the finances for purchasing the products for a complementary protocol.

A daily pattern emerged that seemed to involve the preparation of endless amounts of organic meals, using every available vegetable or fruit, often eaten raw, and the consumption of abundant amounts of vitamin and mineral supplements washed down with gallons of bottled spring water and herbal teas. Juicing was to become one of the main components of my day as most recommendations for holistic cancer treatments suggest including as many fruit and veggie juices as you can.

We are currently on our second centrifugal juicer, which still sees itself subjected to hard labour, grinding such vegetables as sweet potatoes, kale, celery, coriander, cucumber, carrots and raw beetroot. Fortunately, Richard became committed to this organic approach to eating and especially enjoyed the juices and meals prepared with raw food, although I didn't encourage him to give up red meat, as I have done.

Raw food is alive with enzymes, which will not be destroyed through cooking. These enzymes provide the individual with more energy and the assimilation of numerous nutrients, which we know are often lost in processed and cooked food. The idea of including as much as eighty percent raw food in your diet will only improve the body's overall well being and support the immune-system in fighting numerous diseases such as high-blood pressure, cancer and viral infections. The added value that a raw-food diet provides is that it is far less costly on the environment. There are many interesting and comprehensive books on the subject of raw nutrition which should be consulted when considering incorporating a raw food diet into one's life.

CHAPTER 9

FINAL RESULTS

THE day was fast approaching for our visit to the clinic to obtain the results from the tests that had been carried out as a result of my bi-lateral mastectomy. Our nerves were starting to get the better of us and, as Paula had returned to the UK, we no longer had our beautiful grandson as a distraction. During our daily walks, which I insisted we try to carry out most days, we would broach the subject of the worst case scenario that the cancer had spread to other parts of my body. Once again, I would oscillate between the possibility and the impossibility of this happening because, I reasoned, if metastasis had occurred, the strict regime I had put myself on would kill all the diseased cells in my body. Another area we continually discussed was whether I would have the chemotherapy if it was recommended.

On entering the surgeon's office to receive my final results, he greeted us warmly and I was asked to remove my clothes so that he could examine me. By this time I was becoming used to looking down at my ugly frame to where my forlorn breasts had once been and I had no need to feel embarrassed with the doctor as he was so gentle and kind.

He felt all along the scar and proceeded to probe a

couple of areas which, although I had not noticed (I only looked down when it was really necessary and I was still avoiding mirrors when I was naked), were looking very puffy and red. He explained that he would need to aspirate these areas as fluid had collected and it was important not to allow this to continue. Asking the nurse to help him while he drained the fluid, I tried not to appear nervous and, fortunately, it was soon over.

I was told that I must return if this swelling recurred in the future and I have since learnt that this puffiness is called a seroma which is a collection of serous fluid in the area of a wound that sometimes develops in the body after surgery as a result of the incision. When small blood vessels are ruptured, blood seroma can seep out. Inflammation caused by dying, injured cells also contributes to the fluid.

As we had still not been given any final results from the tests of the operation, I broached the subject.

Disappointingly, only half of the results had been completed and it would be another few days before he had the comprehensive report. The doctor could see from our faces that Richard and I were both very frustrated by the lack of information and gave us the details he had received back from the pathologist.

Evidence so far suggested that the cancer had probably taken eighteen months to two years to grow to the size it was and, fortunately, it was analysed as being the type of cancer known as ductal carcinoma in situ (DCIS), oestrogen receptive, Cerp-B2 negative. This appeared to be a positive point as the cancer could be treated with a hormonal drug, such as Tamoxifen, that would act as an oestrogen-blocker. The drug would inhibit the activity of regular oestrogens which simplistically stimulates the division of breast cells, healthy ones as well as potentially cancerous ones. By taking this drug for five years, it would significantly reduce my chances of the cancer returning. During surgery, fourteen lymph nodes had been removed and the biopsy of the left breast (the non-cancerous one) had shown there were various changes occurring.

Although this was positive news, I still did not know whether I would need a course of chemotherapy as this would, in part, depend on whether there was evidence of metastasis (spreading of the cancer) in the lymph nodes that had been removed. We arranged to return the following week to receive the remainder of the report and I suggested to Richard that it would be a good idea if we asked Luisa, our Spanish friend, to attend with us. The more information I was accumulating, the more I formulated questions in my mind, and we may need an interpreter.

The week that followed seemed to be the longest week of my life as, on my dark days, I was convinced that the cancer had spread. However, in the main, I tried to stay positive and continue with my proactive health regime. I was especially excited about one particular part of my complementary treatment plan that I had recently started, which I was sure would cure me. It was simple to prepare, tasted ok and didn't cost very much.

I had discovered the treatment initially from Bill Henderson's book and had also come across it many times during my marathon reading sessions on cures for cancer.

It was a protocol devised by an eminent Physician, Dr Johanna Budwig. She was born in Germany in 1908 and died at the age of ninety-five, having been nominated six times for a Nobel Prize. A top European Cancer Research Scientist, Biochemist, Blood Specialist, Pharmacologist and Physicist, she became a leading authority on the role that fats and oils play in the health of a human body.

As details of her recommendations had occurred time and time again in other literature I had read on complementary treatments for cancer, I decided to carry out extensive research into her background and the rationale behind her rather unorthodox treatment. This is one of the articles describing her work (http://home.online.no/~dusan/diseases/cancer/cancer_dr_budwig.html):

"The Flaxseed (Linseed) oil diet was originally proposed by Dr. Johanna Budwig, a German biochemist and expert on fats and oils, in 1951 and recently re-examined by Dr. Dan C. Roehm M.D. FACP (Oncologist and former cardiologist) in 1990. Dr. Roehm claims: "this diet is far and away the most successful anti-cancer diet in the world".

Dr. Budwig claims that the diet is both a preventative and a curative. She says the absence of linol-acids (in the average Western diet) is responsible for the production of oxydase, which induces cancer growth and is the cause of many other chronic disorders.

The beneficial oxydase ferments are destroyed by heating or boiling oils in foods, and by nitrates used for preserving meat, etc.

The theory is: the use of oxygen in the organism can be stimulated by protein compounds of sulphuric content, which make oils water-soluble and which is present in cheese, nuts, onion leek, chive, onion and garlic and especially cottage cheese."

The above quotation is a simplistic explanation of the complex theory that was studied by Dr Budwig and her team.

The recommended treatment is so simple to implement and I decided to include it within my protocol. Once again there was no immediate proof that the suggested diet of cottage cheese and linseed oil would cure my cancer and prevent it from returning but I felt I had nothing to lose by adding it to my daily diet. Richard religiously prepared the concoction for me and now it is a daily part of our life as a preventative adjunct to our health regime. See Part 2 for further details.

A week later, I was, once again, sitting across from the surgeon, in between Richard and Luisa, who were each holding one of my hands. I leaned forward in anticipation of the final results. Sensing my anxiety, the surgeon launched into the prognosis: fourteen lymph nodes had been removed and there was no evidence of metastasis.

Tears of relief immediately sprang to my eyes as I muttered, "Gracias" and "Thank you", and Richard and Luisa hugged me. It was as good a prognosis as he was able to give me, although he said that he wasn't sure whether the Oncologist, to whom he was referring me, would recommend a course of chemotherapy or just prescribe Tamoxifen for five years.

By this stage, in my understanding of the development of cancer, I appreciated that sometimes rogue cells can escape, even though at the time there may be no evidence of this occurring within one's lymph nodes. Using chemotherapy to mop up the escapees seemed to be a sensible plan of attack. The side effects of Chemotherapy frightened me and still do and I knew that I would have to spend more time getting my head around what I was letting myself in for and look for ways to minimise the fallout from the drug.

Usually, there was at least one month's break before treatment commenced and, therefore, I had plenty of time to do my research! First things first, an appointment needed to be made with the recommended oncologist in Malaga.

More gratitude was expressed as we said our goodbyes to my Spanish surgeon and he gave me a few tips on diet, recommending that I restrict my intake of meat and, when I asked him if soya products were a good substitute, he advised against this also. Apparently, I was to try not to ingest any substance that would encourage my oestrogen levels to increase. He also reassured me that, if there was anything that worried me in the future, I should contact him.

CHAPTER 10

CHANCES OF SURVIVAL

BY the following week I had my first appointment with the Oncologist, a rather handsome doctor in his mid-forties. I knew nothing about him, only that my surgeon had told me that he was highly respected and was one of the top cancer specialists in the country.

It seemed to be the norm, within the cancer medical-field, that there are various specialists that treat the patient, all having specific responsibilities. The UK Consultant that I saw for a second opinion confirmed this by explaining the roles within the team of professionals: a surgeon, an anaesthetist, an oncologist and a radiologist, all of whom would provide the best diagnosis, treatment plan and ongoing care designed specifically around the individual. Spain proved to be no exception, so here I was handing myself over to another expert who would monitor the next stage in my orthodox treatment plan.

The appointment had been scheduled for the evening and I needed to make sure that results of the blood tests that would be required for every visit and were taken at the hospital in the morning would be available on time. On arrival at the modern clinic, I immediately confirmed with the receptionist that she had received them and, handing her my notes, we were invited to sit down in the waiting area.

Conscious that I was surrounded by several people, mainly women, all showing various degrees of sickness, I lowered my eyes and tried not to stare. I failed miserably and as I scanned the scene before me I felt the rock that seemed, during this period of my life, to present itself, when I became nervous, suddenly materialise in the pit of my stomach. This heavy feeling had first become apparent when I was diagnosed with cancer.

A deep empathy with these women accompanied this sinking sensation as all of them seemed to bear the same soulless demeanour. Surveying the surreal scene before me I realised that some were wearing wigs, some were in the throws of re-growing their hair and a few, who looked more 'normal' were, perhaps, attending the clinic for ongoing checkups. All of them, without exception, displayed a grey pallor and slightly swollen faces which looked to me like water retention. I remember thinking that perhaps this was one of the side effects of the drugs.

Picking up a Spanish magazine that was on the table, I attempted to read, but I couldn't concentrate. The words were just a blur. Suddenly I was conscious that a stout lady and a tall man had arrived and settled themselves on the sofa opposite. I felt their eyes on me and I shifted awkwardly in my seat, trying to adjust my corduroy jacket so that my completely flat chest was not too conspicuous.

I had surprised myself as to how, on the surface, I had quickly adjusted to the demise of my breasts. I was so grateful to be alive and to be given the chance to remain alive, in the early days, that I rarely questioned what I looked like. Richard was so stoical and never demonstrated that he felt embarrassed for me or himself, treating me as he always did with love, respect and continually showing me that he still desired me physically.

Demonstrating a typically English trait, I tried to ignore them. Anyone that knows me would agree that I am, by nature, a social character. However, over the past few weeks, neither Richard nor I had felt particularly like socialising. We found ourselves retreating into a world of medical jargon, unorthodox cures for cancer, visits to the local health shops and attending a continuing array of appointments at clinics and hospitals. At this particular moment, I certainly didn't feel like talking to a complete stranger, even if they were from our native country.

A hot flush swept over me and I tried to cool myself by glugging back nearly a half a litre of water. It would have been a relief to have removed my jacket. However, this wasn't an option and, once again, I pulled the two sides together in an attempt to hide my disfigurement. I couldn't avoid their eyes any longer and, looking up, the woman, who was probably in her late fifties, asked me if it was my first visit. We entered into conversation, although I noticed her husband wasn't keen to talk, neither was Richard for that matter.

It is bizarre how complete strangers will pour out intimate details of their medical situation to one another and that is exactly what we did. Establishing that her operation had been a lumpectomy and that she would probably be having chemotherapy and radiotherapy, she then proceeded to tell me how her sister had died of breast cancer five years previously.

I certainly did not want to listen to these negative stories and, throughout the first few months, I tried at all costs to avoid any mention of the fate of individuals who had succumbed to this dreadful disease. I desperately wanted to stay focused on remaining positive and believing I was going to survive. To my mind it isn't very helpful to the cancer victim to be reminded of other alternatives to making a full recovery, such as dying, as they have enough to deal with!

I don't know whether it was the discomfort of our husbands' body language or just an intuitive feeling but I found myself saying how hard the whole process of being diagnosed with breast-cancer was on the husbands and the rest of the family. Missing my point entirely, she continued to describe her family, where they all were, what they were all doing and was eventually interrupted by the receptionist calling her in for her appointment. I wished her luck and said I would probably see her at the next visit.

Slowly, the remainder of the patients waiting to see the oncologist dwindled down to just me and I was relieved to be called into his room. "Rather young", I thought. "I hope that he has plenty of experience."

On arrival at the clinic, I had asked his secretary (who, it transpired, was Canadian and, naturally, spoke perfect English) what his background was. I explained that I knew nothing about him and was curious to understand how long he had been practising in this field.

I received short shrift and she seemed amazed that I should dare to question his experience and authority. A medical hierarchy did exist in Spain after all! To date, I had not seen any evidence of such, unlike in the UK, where you still feel that you have to touch your cap when you meet with a medical consultant, despite decades of encouragement of the medical profession to develop a more open, receptive and empathetic manner towards the patient.

The Oncologist's receptionist did, however, reassure me that he was highly competent, highly qualified and highly respected. Satisfied, if not a little taken back, I wondered why she should be so surprised that I, the patient, should enquire as to my doctor's credentials. Despite her reaction, I would always maintain that it is the patient's right to find out about the medical experience of any doctor treating them. It is normal to want to feel confidence in whoever is treating you and to try to be cured by the very best, especially when dealing with a disease such as cancer.

The Oncologist's English was very good and communication between the three of us didn't prove to be too difficult. My first impressions were that he seemed very unassuming, though somewhat tired - it was, after all, the end of the day and he proved very willing to answer all of my questions.

First things first! He needed to examine me. He took me into a side room, where I removed my clothes. Standing there in front of him, I didn't feel particularly embarrassed as his gentle, confident manner was allowing me to put my trust in his expertise. After a thorough massage of my chest area and examination of my neck and underarms, he softly patted my arm and, with a sympathetic smile, he told me to put my clothes back on.

Sitting back down, I proceeded to fire at him the barrage of questions I had been saving for this day: 'How was I healing?', 'Would I need Chemotherapy?', 'Even though there was no evidence that the cancer had spread, how would we know whether any individual cells had escaped?', 'Why was the only available treatment being used to treat Breast Cancer still the same method that they were using forty years ago?', 'What were my chances of survival?', 'What were the side effects of Tamoxifen?', 'Can I eat meat, fish or soya?'.

Looking down at my notes, the list seemed endless. I had been accumulating these questions ever since the first days of the diagnosis. Carrying them around with me, I was determined to get some straight answers. It was not always to be!

His way of answering some of my questions was to explain the statistics of my survival chances, using a computer programme. Looking at my notes, he commenced typing into his computer some details and checking with me if there were any gaps in the information. A few minutes later he had printed out a graph which included a pie chart and two pieces of written text. The details he handed to us gave a prognosis of someone my age with my type of tumour. The statistics showed what would be the likely outcome if I declined chemotherapy and hormone-related treatment, what would happen if I only received chemotherapy or only the recommended oral drug and, finally, my survival rate if I underwent the Chemotherapy and then took the oral drug for five years.

The results based on my particular case study were:

No additional therapy: 36 out of 100 woman relapse during 10 years.

Taking hormonal therapy such as Tamoxifen only: 79 women out of 100 were still alive after 10 years.

Receiving only chemotherapy: 68 women out of 100 were still alive after 10 years.

Combined therapy of Tamoxifen and chemotherapy: 83 women out of 100 were still alive after 10 years.

The statistics were a little surprising as we could see that there was only an extra four per cent chance of survival after ten years if I agreed to sign up to the combined therapy compared with just taking hormone therapy. Initially, I was apprehensive about the combined approach because, considering the short-term and long-term side effects involved with the chemotherapy treatment and taking the drug Tamoxifen, there did not seem to be much more benefit in subjecting my body to both medications.

When I queried this point, Richard sensibly made the wise comment: "Did I want to be one of the four percent of women who did not survive?" I soon realised that it was better to gain as many advantages as I could when dealing with this life-threatening disease.

CHAPTER 11

DECISION TIME

OVERALL, I was pleased with the approach the Oncologist had used to explain my options. Similar to the UK Consultant, he wasn't able to give me a straight answer as to why the orthodox treatment being used today had not changed in forty years, although the dosages and types of drugs have been refined somewhat. It is unfair to say that no progress has been made in the war against cancer since the end of the Second World War, as there are now new treatments and care that are keeping people alive longer and new, exciting anti-cancer drugs that are still in their trial stages.

However, certain cancers are on the increase and I fail to understand why, considering the funding that has gone into cancer research either through the support of Governments worldwide, particularly from within the UK and the USA, and public donations to the many cancer charities, a cure has not been found. A concrete reason why cancer occurs in the first place would be a reasonable starting point! The longer I questioned my Oncologist, the more I realised that I would just have to keep on searching for the answers.

What I didn't fully understand was why I would still need

chemotherapy when my lymph nodes had been removed and there was no sign of metastasis. Once again the doctor was non-committal and told me that any chemotherapy and radiotherapy treatments in my case were a precaution. I reminded him that I didn't need radiotherapy because I had had both breasts removed. This was one of the few times I was grateful for the amputation of both breasts. This would mean that my treatment would be over quite quickly as I only needed four sessions of chemotherapy over a twelve week period. I also wouldn't have to suffer the debilitating side-effects associated with radiotherapy either.

If the chemotherapy was being administered just as a preventative measure, it was obvious that he could give me no guarantees against the cancer returning. My heart sank again as I realised that the medical profession could not or would not confirm that I was cancer-free. That belief was within me, and the need to convince myself that the cancer had left me on the operating table was getting stronger and stronger as I realised that the doctors could only do so much. My life was in my hands and once again I felt the pull of 'do or die'!

The ball was back firmly in my court and although I was a little frightened, it was now necessary to make a decision as to whether we were going to travel the orthodox route alongside complementary therapies.

The good news was that the healing of my scar tissue was going well. You could have fooled me! The jagged pulsing red scarring made me want to throw up every time I looked at it. I kept telling myself that nothing had changed. I was still the same person regardless of my disfigurement and I was lucky to be alive.

The side effects whilst undergoing the chemotherapy treatment were as I had read. I would be given some drugs to alleviate any nausea I encountered and to prevent me from actually vomiting. It was also very likely that I would lose my hair because of one of the drugs that I would receive. The Oncologist told us that, as I seemed reasonably fit, he would start the chemotherapy treatment the following week and his Secretary would give me an appointment.

Once again, everything was happening so quickly that I hadn't had time to discuss the treatment options with Richard. Conscious that it was the end of a long, tiring day for the doctor and we still had a journey of forty miles home, I agreed to the treatment, knowing that if, after discussions with Richard, we decided against travelling the Chemotherapy path, I could cancel my appointment.

There was just one last question for today; 'What could I eat?' I explained to the Oncologist that I had been given conflicting opinions about what diet I should be on and was it alright for me to take vitamin supplements whilst undergoing Chemotherapy? His recommendations were: no meat, no soya, a little fish and mainly vegetables, beans, grains, nuts and fruit - just as I thought and, once again, I was impressed at his reference to diet as a factor in my treatment. Checking out with me what supplements I was currently taking, he felt that they were fine. We all shook hands and I thanked him very much and, as we left the office of this charming man, I felt quite comfortable that he would do the best he could for me.

We were given an appointment by the secretary on our way out and, coincidentally, the first treatment happened to be taking place on the day before our move into our new apartment. I was also handed the details of various suppliers of wigs as she explained to me that, approximately two to three weeks following the first chemotherapy treatment, my hair would start to fall out. My heart sank and, as I thanked her for the cards, always the eternal optimist, I can remember wishfully thinking that maybe I would be different and I would keep my head of hair.

Driving home gave us the opportunity to discuss the pros and cons of having the chemotherapy. I knew that, whatever was decided, there was no question about me not continuing with my complementary route of treatment. I would do everything in my power to try to mitigate the side effects of the chemotherapy. We talked about my fears of the long term effects on my body and the pros and cons surrounding any decision to have nothing to do with the orthodox approach.

As well as coming to terms with the fact that I had to take medication which, in effect, would poison my body and would make me violently sick, make my hair fall out and compromise my immune system, I was harbouring two conflicting views. The first point was, would I live to regret it if I refused the more conventional drugs to fight the cancer and my other feeling was that by using the more orthodox route, would it totally eliminate every cancer cell in my system? Surely, by wiping out my immune system, it was destroying the very resource that my body needed to make me well? Nothing made sense and I was very confused. Richard emphasised that it was my decision.

I agreed to sleep on it, only I didn't actually go to sleep. For the past few years I had been suffering with sleepless nights and refused to take sleeping tablets, using herbal remedies such as passiflora or valerian to counteract my insomnia. I would often find myself wide awake at two or three o'clock in the morning, sometimes until six o'clock. This pattern seemed to be the norm for many people of my age and I accepted this nightly routine.

During the journey through cancer there would be many

nights where I would lie awake, unable to sleep, alone with my terrifying thoughts and fears. I devised a simplistic deep-breathing healing ritual which I implemented when these situations occurred.

Throughout my late twenties and early thirties, I had become interested in Yoga and, although I never quite became a devout follower as I was always too busy rushing around, the benefits of deep breathing had impressed me: enhancing the function of the lymph system, relaxation of the mind and body and its contribution to the body's self-healing properties, to name just a few. Somewhere, I had also read that by putting yourself in a meditative state through visualizing the cancer cells within the body, it was suggested that one could eliminate them through positive thinking. Whenever I found myself wide awake at some unearthly hour, being tormented by my unreasonable thoughts, I would roll over on to my back and commence my deep-breathing.

The night of my first visit to the Oncologist was a good example of how I used this process to calm my mind and body. Ensuring that I was as relaxed and as comfortable as possible and trying desperately not to wake Richard, I pushed myself down into the bed and stretched out my toes as best I could. Slowly and quietly, I inhaled to a count of five and, starting with the very tip of my toes, I visualised every cell that made up the blood within the cells of my feet. I felt the blood running through my veins moving on up to my ankles, then my calves, not forgetting my knees, especially the right one I had injured after I had run the London Marathon in 2005, all the time remembering to hold my breath for five seconds and exhale for five seconds. Feeling the blood and oxygen rippling through every inch of my body and every organ, I would concentrate on destroying the cancer cells and restoring every cell in every organ to optimum health.

Prayer was an important component of what I was trying to do and my deep concentration was used to make contact with God asking Him to help me with my nightly healing process and remembering to thank Him for my cup which I always felt was more than half full.

Whether it worked or not is not something I question. All I know is that it relaxed me deeply, gave me a warm secure glow and took away any immediate worries I had. Often, I was able to roll over and fall asleep and, if I didn't, then I would use my other coping strategy which was to get up and make cup of herbal tea with an oat biscuit!

CHAPTER 12

SOUP AND TEARS OF LAUGHTER

AT long last, we had been given the completion date for attending the notary to finalise the purchase of our newly-built apartment. We both breathed a sigh of relief and Richard commenced organising the date for the delivery of our furniture and the dozens of boxes of personal belongings that had been in storage since March, when we had sold our villa. At least we would be able to occupy our new home for Christmas to accommodate the whole family and my mother who were joining us.

Several friends had offered to help with the moving-in process. Our son was arriving from Qatar, where he was currently working and would prove to be a great help to his father. My best friend, Paula, offered to fly in from Paris, as did our daughter and grandson, all determined to help where they could.

Normally being the self-sufficient couple we are, any offer of help would have been refused, not wanting to put anyone out. Knowing that all the offers would have been from busy people, we would have struggled on as best we could. However, this situation was different and I was fast learning how to say, 'Yes, please, we do need help.' It was just as well that there were so many people to lend a hand, as is nearly always the case when you move home, and especially into a new home, because a catalogue of disasters began to emerge!

The distraction of our fast-approaching moving-in date and the arrival of family to help us allowed me to tuck away the impending chemotherapy appointment. Deep down, I realised that I had decided that I would be attending the recommended course of treatment; I just needed to forget about it for a while to preserve my sanity. I suppose I was hoping that someone or something would pop up and tell me that everything that was happening to me and my family was just a very bad dream.

The acceptance of what fate has dealt you at any given moment in your life, from my experience, seems to evolve over time. With all the circumstances that I have ever found myself in, there has never been a blinding flash of realisation of how to deal with a situation.

I try to get my head around new information, problem solving, confusions and misunderstandings through going over and over the details in my head, talking non-stop to anyone who will listen, usually my family, and through reading about the particular subject and writing down the details and my thoughts.

The acceptance and coming to terms with cancer and what lay ahead of me slowly evolved into the recognition that I was commencing a journey and I had no idea where it would end. I didn't wake up one morning and, bang, Cancer was staring me in the face. It had quietly moved into my life and there was no going back. If it was there to stay for the short term then I realised that I just had to get on with it and indulge in any whingeing when I was in bed alone at night.

This was easier said than done and I would still have my wobbly days. The odd panic attack and emotional outburst would occur unexpectedly, especially when family and friends were being so kind, supplying us with gallons of home-made soup or when I read the many cards and letters that arrived, brimming over with love and support. This only made me more determined to make my journey a success and be around for these wonderful people that I was privileged to have in my life. After all, cancer is no longer a mysterious disease and its interruption in my life would be dealt with as if it was just another problem-solving situation. There was always something proactive I could do to improve my circumstances.

The move went as well as could be expected, considering we didn't have access to a lift for the first six weeks and we were on the third floor! It took seven men, made up of family and friends, plus two removal men, to transport our furniture and belongings up several flights of stairs from the parking garage in the basement. How hard they all worked as I sat on a packing case down in the basement, directing operations. It was the first day following my initial chemotherapy treatment and, by early afternoon, I was feeling rather nauseous and, therefore, was unable to help very much. By lunchtime, the beds were up and all the furniture was placed in the appropriate rooms. It had all become too much for me and, feeling an overwhelming desire to lie horizontally, I politely excused myself and escaped to the rented apartment that we were still using until ours was ready for occupation.

Quickly preparing myself some of the home-made soup, delivered by our reliable friends, I managed to force a little down, despite the nausea making me not feel like eating. Collapsing on to the settee, as I lay there, I can remember thinking, 'So this is what the effects of the chemotherapy are like. One down and only three to go.' I thought back to the previous afternoon and how the actual Chemotherapy process had been quite straightforward. Sitting in one of the many occupied booths connected up to an intravenous-drip, I had managed to commence reading the biography 'Living History' by Hilary Rodham Clinton. I had bought it the year before, when we had enjoyed another delightful holiday in the USA.

No nausea had been experienced after I left the clinic and I didn't feel any after-effects, only a feeling of slight motion sickness, until approximately twenty–four hours later. The effects of each treatment proved to follow a different pattern, all included the nausea and dizziness and I religiously took the preventative medicine against sickness that the Oncologist had given me. By the third session, I became adept at dealing with the waves of sickness. However, the fourth and final treatment proved to be a different matter.

By the afternoon of that first day, following my first treatment, the decision to withdraw from the commotion of the house move proved the appropriate tonic and a couple of hours rest put me back on my feet. Much to the distress of my family, I was able to resume my position as Chief Director of Operations of the unpacking!

When I was able, to stay occupied helped to keep my mind off the effects the treatment was having on me, and my body would soon tell me when I had done too much. This is one of the benefits that I learnt from the cancer journey: not to push myself to the point of exhaustion as I had done so many times in the past and to stop when I became tired.

The first day of the move had achieved a great deal and Paula from Paris arrived to lend another pair of helping hands. It was a real pleasure to see her with our children and grandchild, enjoying the banter that is so often present when our younger son is around. Often I would feel Oliver's presence and we both remarked on how he would have really enjoyed being with us and having a good laugh. I could see it was hard for her at times, but she always was so supportive, putting the needs of her 'invalid' friend first.

During those first few days, I was often ushered out of the kitchen as Paula took over unpacking the boxes of kitchen utensils and little Richard became chef for the three weeks he was there. He didn't even allow me to commis for him, a task I had always undertaken when he arrived home and took over the kitchen. I didn't mind in the slightest as I was just so delighted to be surrounded by them all and Richard had some help in what proved to be an exhausting but efficient move.

I often sat or lay on the bed as both my wonderful daughter and her godmother quizzed me about where I wanted clothes put away or how ornaments or pictures should be displayed. To be honest, from the way I was feeling, I could not have cared less. The value of these worldly goods had paled into insignificance since my operation. Only restoring myself to optimum health and being with my family and friends really mattered to me.

Decision-making was proving difficult and I often wondered whether the Chemotherapy drugs had affected my brain. 'Chemo brain' became a good excuse to use when my fifty-four year old memory failed me.

Little Paula stayed as long as she could but she had a very patient husband to get back to and when we said our tearful goodbyes, I told her how much I loved her and what a wonderful support she had been to me and her father. I didn't like to think of her having to make the journey every couple of weeks, to see me, especially with a young baby, but I did so benefit from their visits and she was such a sensible sounding board. We both knew that, with Christmas two weeks away, there wasn't too long to wait before we were together again.

It was soon time for the other Paula to leave, too, and she had worked so hard trying to ensure our new home was as organised as possible before she left. The main benefit from her visit at this time was an obvious rekindling of a close friendship we had shared up until our mid teens when distance and circumstances had forced us to go our separate ways. The sense of humour, the emotion and memories had all come flooding back and we both knew that in the future, we would always be able to depend on one another for love and support. In our childhood she had shared her family with me and now it was time to share mine with her.

We were soon as organised as we could be, thanks to the team of helpers. Our young Spanish friends had also offered to help, with Luisa being delegated the responsibility of decorating our Christmas tree. I knew I would certainly not be able to manage this task and it would be very important to me to ensure we erected a colourful tree for Louis-John's first Christmas.

Bob (little Richard) and his father worked like Trojans, erecting mirrors, pictures and climbing the three fights of stairs hundreds of times with shopping and water. Our water had been turned off for short while and it happened that, as we were the only ones occupying the block at that time, our water and electricity would be disconnected from time to time, which is why there were no lifts. This was typical of the usual disorganisation of Spanish building practices. Somehow we coped and kept everything in perspective with laughter and bowls of home-made soup.

Chapter 13

Nice Face, Shame About the Wig!

THE many events that took place during the weeks leading up to Christmas 2007 proved to be a welcome relief to the previous month's activities. It was wonderful spending time with our family and getting to know the treasure of a grandson with whom we had been blessed. On more than one occasion, taking over the feeding of him and experiencing his funny little ways and angelic face distracted me from the soul-destroying sickness I was experiencing.

My elder sister and her daughter's family joined us for Christmas and the New Year and all contributed greatly to an atmosphere of normality, which I was desperately trying to recreate. However, there were many signs which would appear unexpectedly to remind me of the reality of my situation.

Whilst showering one morning, I felt a different type of pain which seemed to travel down my rib cage in a strange thin line. As I ran my finger along this protrusion, I noticed that the soreness travelled from just below the scar tissue where my left breast had been and ended parallel with my navel. On discovering this extremely thin defined lump, the sensation of a mega-hot flush, which occurred frequently during this time, began to take control of my body. Knowing that breast cancer can recur in your breast area, even if you have had your breasts removed, I tried hard to control the blind panic that was engulfing me and I immediately sought a second opinion from Richard.

Fortunately, my second Chemotherapy appointment with the oncologist was imminent and I would be able to check out with him if there was any cause for alarm. At the appointment, a new doctor examined me, as my usual oncologist was on holiday and I tried to hide my disappointment that I wasn't able to discuss my fears with my original doctor, with whom I had quickly built a trusting relationship. The temporary doctor proved to be just as knowledgeable and expertly examined me. He quickly allayed my fears, explaining that the thin bump was likely to be a tendon which, perhaps, I had pulled by exerting myself too quickly, following the operation. However, he would ensure that my Oncologist would give a second opinion at my next appointment at the end of January.

My reaction to the second dose of Chemotherapy was much the same as the first. It was bearable, with the sickness and dizziness occurring two or three days following the treatment, with a maximum of a week unable to eat very much as the nausea took control of my body. I soon realised that, in order to enable me to cope as well as I could with the poisons that were being pumped around my organs, I needed to develop an approach which would help me to work through the discomfort as smoothly as possible.

The first part of the mornings was not too bad and this was when I carried out my domestic chores, preparing innovative dishes with lovely organic vegetables and trying hard to forget about myself and the physical sensations creeping around my body. However, by the afternoon a sense of foreboding and exhaustion presented itself and I was forced to rest. I disciplined myself to drinking plenty of water, fresh vegetable and fruit juices and eating healthily at every mealtime. I followed practically a vegan diet, determined to help my liver and kidneys process the chemicals as efficiently as possible and reduce any burden they may have to endure from any unnecessary additional toxins that a bad diet would induce. Fortunately the anti-nausea drugs worked well and I was only ever physically sick twice, and that was down to the disgusting taste of one of the complementary remedies I was ingesting at the time!

The evenings proved to be the worst period as, by the end of the day, I would experience chronic indigestion, a rather uncomfortable bloated feeling, with my stomach expanding a great deal and the discomfort travelling around the kidney area. I had difficulty in urinating and, to make matters worse, my face would become bright red as, gradually, an intense heat, different from a hot flush, felt as though it was manifesting itself in my brain. The only action I could take was to climb into bed and pull the covers over my head, knowing that, by the morning, at least the redness and the heat would have dissipated. Tomorrow was another day and one day nearer the end of my treatment!

Chemotherapy proved something of a paradox for me. During my treatment I worked hard to discover ways to minimise the side effects that I knew would be happening inside my body as a result of the toxicity of the chemicals I was ingesting. At night, when I couldn't sleep, during my deep breathing sessions and prayer, I visualised the same chemicals doing their work killing the cancer cells and helping in the process of restoring me to health. It was important for me to remain as positive as I could and believe that all my efforts would culminate in a successful conclusion, although I knew that only time would demonstrate true success for me.

During the first few weeks of my journey through cancer, friends kindly bombarded me with articles, books and contact numbers of people who had had experience with cancer. My first reaction was to ignore any information that was in any way negative and my early irrational fear made me skim a lot of information and focus only on what would help me in my quest to eradicate the cancer. Therefore, when the Oncologist's secretary handed me a card for a hairdresser in Málaga who would assist me in finding a suitable wig when my hair fell out, my first reaction was to ignore this gesture and push to the back of my mind, as far as possible, the thought that I would end up bald! After all I had been pumping myself full of all sorts of supplements and potions to prevent this from happening.

My rational self knew that I could not ignore the fact that, after the first treatment, right in the middle of Christmas, it was highly likely that I would lose my hair. I pushed the card in the drawer and got on with preparing for the festivities.

A couple of days before Christmas day I was having my usual morning shower and hair wash when I noticed strands of hair appearing in the shower tray and on my hands. As I tightly held onto my tresses, the sight and texture brought on a bout of the nervous anxiety I experienced throughout my journey. In my ignorance of this situation I had assumed that I would lose my hair in one fell swoop! I thought to myself that it wasn't very much and perhaps the additional vita-supplements were preventing one of the chemo's side-effects of hair loss from taking a real hold, and this is all I would lose. Over the Christmas period, it came out in small amounts and I managed to hang on to the majority of it until the New Year.

If it wasn't for the fact that, every time I sat down, I deposited copious amounts of hair on the furniture and we were vacuuming up to three times a day to keep up with the trails of hair following behind me, I think I would have been curious to wait and see if I did, in fact, lose all of my hair and, more importantly, to discover whether the recommendations I had taken from the cancer books I was reading did help me retain some of my mane. I was not looking forward to seeing myself bald, wearing a wig or becoming an object for some people to stare at!

The appointment with the wig-fitting salon proved to be as miserable an experience as I had thought it would be. Richard was his usual supportive self and the assistant was professional and charming, obviously used to dealing with sullen cancer patients. I could not muster any enthusiasm and, although I do not feel that I am a particularly vain woman, I was convinced that there was not a wig around that didn't look like a wig and they would all look ridiculous on me. Eventually Richard and the assistant chose a Raquel Welch model and they agreed that, after the wig had been given a wash and a trim, I would look as good as new! I arranged to collect it at the beginning of January when I went for my next Chemotherapy treatment.

Christmas 2007 will always stay etched in my memory as not only the time I was recovering from breast cancer but as an extremely testing period for the family and, at times, the atmosphere was extremely intense. A great deal of worry had been generated through my illness and the anxiety that my children felt did not go unnoticed. The stress Richard had been under obviously was alleviated somewhat by having his family with him. Realising that his father would need a break, his son organised for him to go to a football match in Barcelona, which took them both away for twenty-four hours from the difficult environment they found themselves in. Our daughter appeared to busy herself with her first born, trying to create a normal Christmas environment for everyone, and her husband, exhausted from working hard running his own business, quietly relaxed in the Spanish sunshine, offering support whenever he could.

I sensed that my mother, sister and brother-in-law were still unsure as how to deal with my situation and how to behave around me, and their sadness must have been unbearable at times. The presence of their family's little grandchildren helped and, overall, we all had a reasonable Christmas. Love and care were in abundance and being together was all that mattered.

With the New Year came the new wig, and my relationship with it commenced with a loathing that remained for the duration of its usage. Oh how I hated that wig and everything it represented. Everyone was so kind when confronted with my new hairdo and showered me with lots of compliments: 'I would never have known it was a wig', 'You look so glamorous', 'It's better than your real hair'. My daughter was more honest, stating that I looked like Ann Diamond on a bad hair day!

One positive aspect of wearing a wig was that it cut down considerably the time it takes to get ready when you are going out and only became a real problem if the weather turned windy or I wanted to try on clothes in a shop changing booth. I suppose it wasn't the wig's fault that I hated it so much. The synthetic quality and the attractive short cropped style of the product certainly were of a high standard but our relationship just didn't get off to a very good start. Once I realised that maybe my hair was not going to stop falling out, we returned to the salon for the task of shaving my head.

We arrived slightly late for the appointment and I went ahead whilst Richard parked the car. Have you ever tried sitting in a salon chair and avoid looking at yourself in the mirror? Impossible! I was not relishing the thought of watching what was left of my hair being shaved off. I kept my eyes lowered whilst the hairdresser attacked my hair with such precision and efficiency, and I wondered whether she enjoyed this part of her job.

In five minutes the task was completed and, looking up, I saw a hairless woman with a stubble of fine dark hair covering the surface of her scalp. I pretended it wasn't me and, as the hairdresser positioned the wig on my head and complimented me in Spanish, I tried very hard to smile and make my 'Gracias' sound sincere. Unfortunately, the sight that was before me only added to the resentment that was growing inside me concerning this part of my journey. When I think back to those days now, I wasn't experiencing a feeling of self pity but more a distaste of how I looked.

Every day I had tried to discourage myself from sinking into a self-piteous and self-indulgent state and was grateful for the proactive protocol that was taking me along the road to full health, but I would be lying if I said that it never bothered me to lose my hair and breasts. At times it did, usually when I was in the bathroom or in a passionate embrace with my husband. I know that it was my problem because never once did Richard ever make me feel anything other than special and deep down I knew I was still the same person, just minus boobs and hair.

Disappointed with the black stubble that remained, I quickly understood what a close shave means to a man. I had visualised coming away from the experience with a perfectly formed oval head with a lovely glossy shine!

By the time Richard arrived at the salon to collect me,

the new wig was being styled to suit the shape of my face. He was astonished at how quickly the whole process had taken and couldn't get over how well the wig suited me and matched the colour of my original hair. For a moment, he said he had not recognised the glamorous person sitting in the chair as being me!

On leaving the salon, the first task was to dive into the department store next door to buy a hat to protect the wig from the wind and rain and search for some more Kylie Minogue-style bandanas. I had no intention of wearing the wig indoors unless I was forced to. My sister had managed to send me some scarves made by volunteers in a cancer unit at the local hospital but I felt I would need an abundant supply as they would need washing frequently. At first, the wig made me feel as though I was wearing a hat and was, at times, very hot and claustrophobic. Naturally, it proved useful when it was cold.

After the initial shaving of my head, I was very reluctant to expose my baldness to Richard but I was so disappointed with the protruding black stubble that he offered to give me a close shave. I gritted my teeth praying that he wouldn't nick my scalp and my prayers were answered as Richard successfully removed the unwanted hair as if he was an experienced barber.

Slowly the Raquel wig became part of my outdoor life although, as soon as I set foot indoors, off it came. I would scurry into the bedroom or bathroom, whip off the wig, replacing it with a bandana, which was far more comfortable, trying all the time not to expose my head to Richard or anyone else around at the time. Morning showers were taken before Richard got up and at night the bandana came off when the light went out. One day I was explaining to someone how upsetting the whole baldness and wig business was and Richard emphasised that it didn't bother him at all. An effort was then made on my part to conquer the feelings of embarrassment I was experiencing and integrate my bald head firmly into family life!

Strangely enough the only person I didn't mind seeing my baldness was my son-in-law and that was because, in his younger days, a friend had shaved his head for a joke and he understood how I felt. The children, understandably, stated they were uncomfortable with the thought of a bald-headed mother and, therefore, I never did expose my head in their presence. When my hair started to grow and a respectable crew cut appeared, I discarded the wig, and our grandson would stare at me strangely from time to time, not quite sure whether this was still the same nanny that had been carrying him around since he was a newborn.

CHAPTER 14

ONGOING TREATMENT

CHRISTMAS was soon over and the family returned to the UK to resume their hectic lives and try to put behind them the distress and concerns that they had all inevitably experienced when someone they love is diagnosed with cancer. As we saw them off at the airport, I knew that their lives had been changed by my journey through cancer. The individual relationships I had with each of them would never be the same and they would always view me differently. The experience we had all gone through over the past six weeks had changed each one of us forever. An opportunity had presented itself to us to no longer take life for granted and arrogantly assume that a life-threatening disease would never strike one of us, least of all me, who had prided herself on living a healthy life.

Many times, I had concerned myself about the big C attacking a member of the family as, with all families, mine included several smokers and individuals who didn't pay attention to a healthy diet or how much alcohol they drank.

A point that still concerns me a little is the fatalistic attitude some people have adopted since they heard about my plight. The usual throw-away statements were offered when the subject of 'why me' came up. Such conversations would include remarks such as, 'What is the point of worrying about looking after yourself when life is mapped out for you', 'Enjoy yourself, do what you want to and have whatever you want.'

Although, in principal, I can relate to the concept of not taking life too seriously and it is something I aim to carry out now more frequently, it is my belief that we all have responsibility for our health and well being. It is unwise to leave the fate of your health in the lap of the Gods, after all it is one of the few things we still have control over.

Even if the disease you may acquire is genetic and you are fortunate enough to know this fact, prevention is still better than cure. If all in the Western World took their life style and health more seriously, it certainly would help contribute towards alleviating at least one of the financial burdens of Governments: overburdened and underfunded Health Services.

By the middle of January 2008, I was halfway through my treatment and, with the Raquel wig well and truly installed, I felt I was coping quite well. Some days were better than others and, on my good days, I would get up early and march five kilometres along the promenade whilst Richard carried out his training for the London Marathon. I counted my blessings that I had only needed four sessions of Chemotherapy and no Radiotherapy, which would have prolonged my treatment by another 6 weeks.

Every three weeks, each Chemotherapy session would last between forty minutes and one hour and involved being hooked up to a drip which contained the necessary chemotherapy drugs. The time in between each treatment allowed the drugs to carry out their work and the body to recover somewhat before the next onslaught of medication.

I counted the number of days until the treatment would be finished and I could plan my life once more. The final week of each three week period felt like a paradox as I looked forward to less nausea and a better appetite but dreaded the thought that I would be returning to the clinic for yet another shot of the cancer medication.

Family and friends continued to spur me on with words of encouragement, explaining to me that I only had one or two more treatments and how well I looked and how well I was coping.

What would we have done without these wonderful people, my husband, children and superb grandson? Paula managed to visit regularly with Louis-John, who gave me so much pleasure over the coming weeks, especially during my chemotherapy periods when I felt very low. Watching my eight month-old grandson grow rapidly and experience his funny little ways is an indescribable delight, and his infectious laugh gave me so many moments of pleasurable relief from the heavy cloud that seemed, on occasions, to engulf me. He was a blessing in disguise and I feel so privileged to be part of his life.

Although I really appreciated all of the support, sometimes, however, I couldn't help but think that these well meaning people didn't have a clue what it was like to be in this position and, at times, I felt patronised.

I know this seems unfair and unreasonable and I really regretted snapping at my sister when she tried to make me feel better about my wig by saying that when my hair grew back it would be stronger, thicker and curly. Whilst she was trying to reassure me, I turned and asked her rather curtly, 'How would you have coped with losing your hair?' Being a former hairdresser, her hair is always immaculate and we often pull her leg about the number of hours she spends in the morning perfecting her coiffure! As soon as it came out of my mouth, I knew it was a cruel question and I would not have wished my circumstances on my worst enemy.

I just wanted someone to talk to that hadn't been so painfully affected, someone who could listen to my fears and anxieties without me trying to protect them from any more hurt - someone who had been in the same situation and had come out of the experience with a positive outcome. Often, people were very insensitive when recounting stories of individuals who had succumbed to breast cancer and, at this stage in my journey, I really did not want to hear any negative information.

It was most fortunate that, just before Christmas, I had been introduced to a woman who was in the first year following the end of her treatment for breast cancer. Jenny proved to be an invaluable and sensitive source of help. Always there to listen to my questions and offer advice based on her experiences, she was able to prepare me as to what the next stage would be and how I might feel. She is younger than me by at least ten years and has rebuilt her life, returning to teaching and her role as a ballroom-dance instructor.

Jenny was able to give me advice about the effects of the Chemotherapy treatment. She warned me that the third treatment may be the hardest to tolerate and the fourth not so bad. This surprised me as I had thought that, as each treatment kicked in, the body would find it more and more difficult to withstand the side effects and the fourth would surely be the worst.

The first treatment had not been as bad as I had envisaged, which was just as well, what with our house move two days after the visit to the clinic. The main side effect involved an overwhelming sense of seasickness which descended on me and relief would only come if I lay horizontally and tried to sleep.

A strange experience occurred when I arrived home from the hospital, following the second treatment. We were climbing the several flights of stairs because the lifts were still not working and, as I reached the top, the most excruciating pain passed through my lower back. It felt as though I had been stabbed and, for a few minutes, I couldn't walk and was convinced that terrible damage had been done to my kidneys. Hurrying into the house, I drank a large quantity of water, hoping that this would flush out my kidneys. For twenty-four hours, following each treatment, my urine was a bright red colour due to the type of drug I was ingesting. Therefore, I knew the importance of taking in copious amounts of fluid.

Apart from this peculiar incident, memories of the effects of the second treatment seem to have been overshadowed by the episode of losing my hair and carrying out the usual settling-in process involved with a house move. However, I was not looking forward to treatment number three and I was certainly unprepared for the effects that I experienced on day four. Standing at the sink, preparing, as usual, the organic vegetables for the day's meals, the seasickness kicked in with such ferocity that I thought I might pass out. So as not to panic Richard, who was assembling a kitchen cupboard, I crept into the lounge and lay on the sofa. There I stayed to await a lull in the symptoms which would enable me to perhaps prepare some lunch. The respite didn't arrive and I was forced to stay horizontally glued to the sofa for the rest of the day.

Weakness crept over me and robbed me of my power of speech and any motivation to physically move around just ebbed away. Stretched out on the sofa in a rigid parallel posture I had been compelled to create, I can only describe that the paralysis was accompanied by a sense of the light within my soul fading. This dramatic sensation of my life-force diminishing had shown itself previously during the treatment and was quite different from any form of depression or sadness I had encountered in my life to date. It stealthily crept through my body attacking my mind and draining me of any enthusiasm for day-to-day living. As the treatment robbed my body of the motivation to live, a battle of wills ensued as I became weaker and weaker as I felt I was drawing on my last ounces of strength and resolve to ensure I did not let go of my will to live. Many times, I wondered what the optimum number of treatments that a patient could tolerate may be. I was so grateful mine would end at four and prayed that the final one would not be so bad.

I never thought that Julie Andrews would come to my rescue that day as I lay there devoid of all feelings and sensations, but she did. My nephew had sent me some DVDs and amongst them was the epic version of The Sound of Music. Although incapable of much conversation or expression, I found that I was capable of mentally interacting with the characters in the Sound Of Music and it certainly filled the five hours that I was feeling very poorly.

The experience during the fourth treatment was equally as bad but, by now, I had learnt certain coping mechanisms for alleviating the symptoms. The good days reminded me that this state was only temporary and it would not be long before I was on the road to recovery.

CHAPTER 15

COMPLEMENTARY PROTOCOL

DURING my quest for complementary remedies, my homoeopathist recommended to me an EFT practitioner who also happened to be a qualified counsellor. EFT is a very effective yet gentle method of directly balancing the body's energy system for the feelings that you want to change. It's a bit like clearing a log that's blocking a stream where the log represents a stuck emotion in your stream of energy. You don't have to believe in the theory though, just as you don't need to know how a car works under the bonnet to drive one.

Using EFT involves 'tuning into' the issue and then tapping with your fingers on specific acupressure points with your fingers. For example, if you still carry anger towards someone who has hurt you in the past, you would be asked to think about them, and notice how you feel. But you do not have to relive past events. You just have to be aware that the negative feeling is there. Having, therefore, 'tuned in' to it, you are shown which acupressure points to tap, and what words to say as you do so. (Saying a few things also helps to disperse the emotion from the system).

Having carried that out, you are then asked to think

about the person or situation again and check how you feel. Typically, you will notice a significant reduction in the intensity of the feeling. If it's not completely gone then the EFT practitioner repeats the process, bringing the intensity down each time until full balance is restored.

Always open to new ideas and holistic practices, I listened intently as the explanation was given as to what my role would be when practising the technique. The first step was to establish a life-changing statement. During my meetings with the EPT instructor, I had been reluctant to enter into any counselling sessions. I knew from the counselling experience that I had had when John died that it would require total commitment from me in both time and energy and I did not feel, at that stage in my life, that I could, with everything that was going on, dedicate myself wholeheartedly to the process. I was also concerned that a can of worms would be opened up about my life and my shattered nerves, at this stage, could not begin dealing with any more exploding emotions.

From my perspective, counselling can be an enlightening experience, offering the patient an insight into the darkness of their problems and often how to discover a solution to those problems. This can only be achieved when the individual demonstrates total openness and a degree of being true to oneself. For all my reluctance to refrain from entering into a counselling session at this stage of my journey, I soon realised that taking part in EFT would need me to open up a little as to how I was coping.

With total honesty, I explained to the Counsellor that this was not the time or place to address too many issues as I didn't want to become bogged down with my past personal problems when trying to deal with my journey through cancer. She was extremely helpful and understanding and we agreed that maybe at a later date, when I was further down the road of recovery, I could pick up some therapy along the way.

Although we did try very hard to focus on the practical side of the EFT healing, it was soon necessary for me to reveal some insight into my feelings, emotions and views about my journey. We touched on subjects such as the effect of the operation on my sexuality, Richard's support and views, my two-pronged orthodox and complementary attack on the disease, how my family were coping, what role my father played in my life, the relationship I had with my mother, siblings and children, a little about my childhood, losing John and Oliver and the other bereavements I had encountered in 2007.

These subjects evolved out of the part of the EFT process that required me to write down several affirmations that I would like to change about myself and in my life. It soon became evident from the above topics of discussion that my main statement would begin: *'Even though I don't always achieve what I want to in a day,'* and it was very important to always end the statement: *'...I truly and profoundly accept myself'*.

Understanding the concept of EFT was easy but carrying out the ritual was another thing entirely. However, every day I would religiously carry out the chanting of the affirmation and tapping, disciplining myself to lie or sit down whilst I performed the task. The areas of tapping on the body correspond to certain chakra points and it was very important to concentrate and not to let your mind wander because, for one thing, you would forget what number you were up to with your tapping or you would lose the sense of the sentence as your thoughts drifted off to think about the shopping or what food needed to be prepared for dinner!

As the days went by, I stopped feeling silly when I was in my tapping trance-like state, almost welcoming the time I spent lying on the bed, dedicating myself to being the focus of attention in a structured, positive way. On one particular occasion it was early evening and Richard had gone on an errand, so I decided to carry out my chanting. It was at the end of the day and I really did not feel like making the effort, but a little voice egged me on and I positioned myself on the sofa. Towards the end of my chanting I felt a strong desire to fall forward on my knees and pray out loud. With my hands stretched up like a mad woman, I faced the sea and sky and I gave thanks to God for my health and happiness, for helping me through the dark times. Drawing my arms to me and then opening them out towards the sky I prayed that He allow his light and love to enter into me and may it continue to give me strength to cope with life, that He looked after all my family and friends, keeping them safe, and I finished off the prayer by asking Him to bless the world.

All I can say about the tremendous energy and feeling of hope that filled me at this time is that it truly felt like the power of God. Whether the chanting acted as a catalyst for this experience, I don't know. All I can do is explain just how it happened.

Another fundamental change that happened during this period of practising EFT was that, instead of trying to fit a hundred and one activities into the day and beating myself up if I didn't achieve them, I was more relaxed and laid back, realising that tomorrow really was another day and what wasn't achieved that day really was no big deal. My new approach to organising my life enhanced the great periods of mental well-being, contentment and happiness that I was experiencing from time to time. This was, I am sure, partly due to a new appreciation of life, having found myself in a vulnerable position where my life had been threatened, and the power of positive prayer. The holistic organic diet was also having a profound affect on my constitution and personality moods.

CHAPTER 16

CROSSROADS

THE final chemotherapy treatment day arrived and everyone was ecstatic for me. The very thought of not ever having to have any more chemotherapy made the dose almost bearable. I say almost as, by this time, I recognised that my bright days, when I felt relatively normal, were becoming less frequent. This, I am sure was down to the chemicals accumulating in my cells, tissues and organs, affecting my whole being. My skin had taken on the grey pallor that I had observed on the other patients in the waiting room when I had first met the Oncologist. Fortunately, I had only lost two kilos in weight and, having read that it is advisable not to lose more than 3 kilos, I counted myself fortunate.

There were also days, in between treatments, where the sensations of extreme well-being kicked in and the thought of carrying out such a task as climbing Everest seemed a possibility! I could only put this down to the body's defence mechanism winning the fight against the disease and the negative effects of the chemotherapy. However, these occasions were becoming less frequent.

No amount of times being reminded that it was the final treatment seemed to raise my spirits during the days prior to my last chemotherapy session. Mentally, it was the lowest I had felt all the way through my journey so far. The side effects were not any worse than I had previously experienced; it just seemed that my body was telling me it was getting to the point that it had had enough of being attacked. The regular blood tests highlighted that my immune system was struggling to recover.

The first blood test I received, following my final chemotherapy, proved to be interesting as it revealed that my white blood count was fifty per cent below the minimum normal range. Simplistically, the white blood cells, which are made up of several different types of cell, all having an important function in the fight against disease, were struggling to recover to an acceptable level. Like me, they obviously had very little resilience left and I knew there was a lot of work to be done to improve my natural defence mechanism. I thought about a nasty throat infection that had occurred after Christmas. It had been responsible for my temperature reaching a critical level of 37.5°C and the worry that this had caused Richard because he knew that the oncology clinic had given us strict instructions that if my temperature reached 38°C I should be admitted to hospital immediately.

My susceptibility to infection, on balance, was probably no worse or no better than anyone else in my position and, as my body was continuing to ward off many infections, sore throats, coughs and the mouth ulcers which continuously plagued me, I was anxious to commence, as soon as possible, a more comprehensive immune-system building regime.

With my orthodox protocol drawing to an end, I wondered where my journey would take me next. I realised I had

118

arrived at a crossroads and needed to make a decision as to which path I should take to achieve my next objective. In reaching my ultimate goal, which was the light at the end of the tunnel, I had finally come to terms with the fact that the completion of my chemotherapy was not an end in itself.

Just prior to the final session of Chemotherapy in February, 2008, Richard and I decided to attend a presentation, further down the coast, on alternative and complementary therapies. The details had been given to me by the owner of the health shop that I was using at the time to buy my supplements. Coincidentally, I had read a reference to the Clinic based in Marbella, delivering the presentation, in the book, "Healing Cancer Gently", by Bill Henderson, that we had downloaded from the internet in the previous November.

The venue was somewhat of a surprise as the guest speakers delivered their information in the living room of the organiser's apartment in order to keep the cost down for the attendees. The two men, one of whom was a reporter for a local magazine, and responsible for the planning of the evening, explained his role as a catalyst for bringing together experts who could offer information and knowledge on treatments for cancer, heart disease, diabetes, etc.

The speaker who was representing the clinic proved to be an interesting character who demonstrated to the group of twenty people, crammed into the apartment, that he was very knowledgeable in the field of complementary therapy. His talk, which lasted approximately one hour, didn't waver in presenting the facts of how the human-body can heal itself with the help of a healthy protocol consisting solely of complementary holistic therapies. He expounded many theories, mentioning such people as the famous scientist,

Dr Budwig, and impressed us with his ability to tackle a number of controversial questions which were thrown at him by the listeners. The audience consisted of people of different ages and from all walks of life. Some of the individuals who suffered or had suffered from various terminal diseases had travelled quite a distance to hear the presentation. I could relate to the urgency of their quest to find help to cure themselves.

One area that the presenter was very dogmatic about was the use of chemotherapy in the treatment of cancer. His criticisms and general abhorrence of this Western orthodox protocol annoyed me somewhat and, as I tried to be objective about his comments, I found myself thinking that perhaps I could have been cured without resorting to such dramatic measures as bombarding myself with man-made chemicals.

He described the billion-dollar pharmaceutical industry, which was responsible for producing the drugs that undoubtedly poison the healthy cells as well as attacking the cancer cells, as being giant corporations that had little intention of proactively finding a natural non-destructive cure for cancer. Their only objective seemed to be of self-interest and to expand distribution and improve the chemicals that were helping to lubricate such a successful money-making machine.

I couldn't subscribe to all that he expounded at this stage in the presentation. However, perhaps there was a degree of truth in some of his views. Whenever I wavered from believing that I had taken the appropriate course of action regarding the orthodox treatment I was receiving, I tried to hang onto the fact that there are thousands of successful cases of individuals who have undergone chemotherapy and survived.

At the end of the presentation, a promotional financial discount was offered to anyone who was interested in receiving a comprehensive physical analysis and details were given of the various health assessments available, using all sorts of techniques and equipment. I decided, there and then, that I wanted to arrange an appointment with the clinic and find out exactly what they could add to my own protocol that had been evolving over the last few weeks. As usual, when I asked Richard his thoughts, he was supportive and went along with whatever I proposed. Sometimes, I would detect some concerns from him as to how many more supplements, potions or treatments I would be trying!

It really was trial and error and I desperately needed evidence, if not for myself then for the people around me who were watching the drastic changes I was making to my lifestyle. I had always had what some people deemed to be a rather bizarre and obsessive approach to health, believing emphatically in the 2.5 litres of water per day rule and carrying, without failure, the elixir of good health around in a plastic bottle wherever I went!

I would bore nearly everyone almost to tears with my commitment to a low-fat, almost meat-free diet and abundant amounts of vegetables and exercise. I say nearly everyone because there were people who appreciated my lecturing on the virtues of taking responsibility for one's own health and fitness. There were times when I would lapse, of course, and would binge on chocolate, cakes and alcohol. By binge, I mean two glasses of red wine as, when I reached my late forties, this was usually sufficient for my physical constitution!

There was no way of knowing whether any of the complementary health substances I was taking were having an effect on the cancer, or the chemotherapy, for that matter. I just had to believe that all the efforts being carried out were working. An appointment with the clinic in Marbella was made and the first question I wanted answered would be how I could measure to what degree my self-devised protocol was improving my health?

Once again, I gave myself over to another individual who I believed would help me build my body back to optimum health and move me along the road to recovery. The conviction that my own body was the only tool that could truly heal me was growing stronger. Although I knew that it would need all the help it could receive, niggling doubts still came into my mind from time to time that the decision to have the chemotherapy had only added to the pressure my little body was under!

CHAPTER 17

A LONG WAY TO GO

AT my first appointment with the new clinic, the therapist explained to me that the starting point would be a comprehensive blood test which would detail almost every aspect of information related to the functioning of my organs, heart, liver, kidneys, pancreas, red and white blood cells, iron and potassium levels etc.

He showed me a completed blood test of someone in peak condition and several items were highlighted as pointers to optimum health such as: Alkaline Phosphatase (a detector of liver disease or bone disorders), Total Bilirubin levels (another test for liver disorders) and Lactic Dehydrogenase (to identify the cause and location of tissue damage in the body). Though this medical jargon was double Dutch to me, I was glad of the information and, following every appointment, I would scour the Internet, searching for an understanding of the terminology my new therapist was using.

It appears that all of the test results in Spain become the property of the patient and it was the norm for my consultant to hand over any documentation, following the consultation process, to me. Therefore, when I received the details of the blood test that my oncologist used during my six-monthly check-ups, I would compare the results with the new blood test I was receiving during my complementary treatment and with the sample blood test I had been given by the therapist of someone in peak condition.

The hospitals and laboratories I used in Spain seemed to have slightly different ranges for describing a normal blood test and it was explained to me that the median they use is that of an average individual. Therefore, these measurements will show the blood of a relatively well person but not someone in peak condition. Although, as the weeks went by, I realised my blood would never be as good as an elite athlete, I understood the benefits of using the blood test with superlative markers as a motivator for improving my health.

The therapist continued to stress what tasks were involved in the treatment and I soon recognised that his objective was to ensure that, through monitoring the markers within the blood of every individual he treated, he was able to determine to what level the quality of their blood was steadily improving. These changes in the blood would be achieved through diet, various treatments and supplements. The knowledge and expertise he had were impressive. The Clinic had been established for a long time and the founder appeared to be medically well-qualified. However, I never saw evidence that my particular therapist had acquired any academic qualifications and, when this worried Richard or myself, I pacified us by stressing that I had never seen any formal qualification structure for the complementary health industry - only on-the-job experience.

Using the results of the ideal blood test, the therapist explained the details of what each recorded component related to. For example, which abbreviation or symbol represented the level of iron in my body or how to read a low blood count. I soon became very apt at analysing my own blood tests. I am sure there would be some medical practitioners who, when reading my previous comment, would throw their hands up in horror at the thought of a lay person, not medically-trained, reading their own blood tests. All I can say is that, once I rid myself of the anxiety of the responsibility that having access to such important information about myself entailed, I was able to utilise it proactively and see how the results could help me to understand how to improve my well being

In time, owning this data about the condition of my state of health made me feel liberated, in control of my disease and reinforced my desire to take responsibility for healing myself. This approach may not work for everyone and that is why it is important to work alongside very competent health and medical practitioners and not rely totally on your own judgement and instinct.

Using information from the first of the four blood tests I had received at the recommended clinic, my protocol was quickly devised by my new practitioner and at the core of the pattern of treatment was the regular suggestion of fortnightly liver flushes. Although I carried them out like an obedient client, my body never ever felt comfortable with the process, although I am sure they successfully completed their objective which was to rid the liver of any toxins, parasites and, more importantly, any residual chemicals which may be lurking there.

Alongside this treatment, I had decided to subject my bowel to further cleansing in the form of weekly colonic irrigation for the time I was undergoing chemotherapy. I had read that this would help rid the bowel of any toxins that maybe ingested back into the bloodstream.

The mountain of locally-grown organic vegetables, fruit and daily doses of rice bran certainly helped to keep my digestive tract clean and I only once suffered from the chronic constipation that sometimes afflicts chemotherapy patients. Regular lymphatic drainage massages, I am sure, also helped and allowed me an opportunity to relax in very pleasant surroundings.

Following the Health Practitioner analysis of my blood test, using the pro-forma that he had requested the clinic to carry out, I was sent a report which identified twenty-two problems. Understandably, the biggest area to tackle was a severe viral infection which, combined with a weak immune system, was hindering my recovery.

No time was lost in taking on board the recommendations in the report and, by my next blood test four weeks later, my white blood cells had improved by fifty per cent and the ratio increase of the neutrophils (white blood cells which can find and kill bacteria and other infectious organisms) and lymphocytes (immune response white blood cells in the bone marrow) was going in the right direction. By the following month, due, I believe, to an additional recommendation sent to me by the therapist, which I readily adopted, my white cells increased by another fifty per cent, surpassing the healthy range for the optimum blood test. I was delighted and, by the end of April, any previous reference to Neutropenia, a condition which often occurs as a result of chemotherapy, had disappeared. I continued with the fortnightly liver flushes and some of the short-term supplements were discontinued by the time I was scheduled to see the oncologist for my six monthly check.

Before my first check up, following the end of the chemotherapy, a welcome trip to the UK, for Richard to run the London Marathon in aid of Breast Cancer Campaign, proved to be just what the doctor ordered.

It was a great opportunity to be together as a family with our son joining us from Qatar. Richard successfully completed the marathon in four hours twenty eight minutes, one of his best run times - not bad for a fifty-six year old, who had taken the role as the carer of a cancer sufferer throughout his training period. He attributes how well he recovered from the marathon to the diet, juicing and supplements we were both taking and, as an added bonus, raised three thousand, seven hundred and eighty pounds for the charity. The money was raised in the main by the family holding various funding raising functions and our friends on the Costa del Sol organizing barbecues, etc.

We returned to Spain, both uplifted from spending time with the family and the success of the London Marathon, to prepare for a holiday in the USA and for my six-monthly check with the oncologist. The blood test for the oncologist, taken two weeks following the one that showed a marked improvement in my overall health, proved to be a disappointment as it showed that my white cells had decreased by fifty percent and Neutropenia had returned. The dramatic change in my blood test in two weeks demonstrated for me that the short-term supplements that I had been taking and the recommendations from the therapist, during the month of April, needed to be continued for a longer period as there was no way my body had fully recovered. Residual chemicals from the chemotherapy were still festering in my cells.

On reflection, a year down the road of recovery, the results of the five blood tests interestingly showed that, from the time of my final chemotherapy in February until the end of May, the number of white cells had steadily increased. My red cell count, although slightly below the normal range, did not vary very much, despite efforts to improve the situation. At my first six-monthly check, my oncologist made reference to this fact by observing that my red blood cells were taking a time to recover.

Everything always seems different in hindsight. However, at the time, I was bitterly disappointed and, realising that I had been naive to believe that, once the chemotherapy had finished, my body would return immediately to normal, I continued my journey along the slow road of recovery. At no time did I consider asking the question of how long it would take to rid my cells of the residual chemicals. I knew that the answer would be that it depends, as everyone will recover differently.

Patience is a virtue and a virtue I have never had very much of and, during the remainder of the year, it would be tried time and time again. Maybe this was the biggest lesson I would need to learn: that I had to accept that my body was an organism which needed nurturing over a period of time and could not be bullied into a complete recovery as and when I demanded!

There was also the other consideration, which was that this journey of recovery was being managed by me a lay person when it came to understanding complementary therapies. Although, so far, I had had a great deal of excellent help and advice from the complementary therapists, I felt that I had yet to hit on the jackpot cure, if there was one! When the negative doubts crept into my mind as to whether any of the remedies I was ingesting were working, I counteracted these thoughts with the fact that the chemotherapy may have offered a lot more horrific symptoms if I had not followed the holistic path alongside the orthodox route.

The Complementary therapist continued to tackle the problem of decreasing white cells over the next two weeks and, at the end of May, with our American summer holiday looming, I had to resign myself to the fact that the following six months, until my next meeting with the Oncologist, would be an opportunity to move on to the next stage of my recovery and to see where the journey through cancer would lead me. Armed with my liver flush instructions and various vitamin supplements, we flew to Florida!

CHAPTER 18

LYMPHOEDEMA AND ROCK AND ROLL

PROBABLY the biggest paradox that I encountered on my journey, during the first year of my recovery, was that despite the abundance of valuable information on cancer, within both the complementary and orthodox fields of health, covering such areas as surgical, medical, adjunctive therapies, physiotherapy, spiritual, emotional, nutritional and helping strategies to cope with the disease, there always seemed to be an opportunity to miss some vital information.

Whether that was due, in part, to my own intellect, failing to absorb all of the facts correctly or the information not being presented appropriately in the first place, I will never know. However, a lesson I have learnt is to ensure that, as far as possible, you should try to manage the interconnectedness of all of the details on cancer that you receive either through your own research or through well-meaning individuals passing on information. Don't take anything for granted and glean as much information as you possibly can from the medical profession by asking questions. It was this issue that prompted me to design a mind map for the second part of my book.

Often, cohesiveness of the patient's healing protocol does not play a part in the recovery of the individual; sometimes it can appear very much hit and miss. There could be several reasons that this occurs, one of which is that, occasionally, the patient does not pay attention to the detail of their condition and forthcoming treatment, blindly following the Doctor's orders. When one considers the enormity of what they may perceive before them, it is not surprising. Another reason could be that the patient and their family simply have not been told all the facts and the detail of what their contribution is to their recovery.

Information concerning cancer was fast flowing in all sorts of formats from very well-meaning friends and family during the first few weeks of my diagnosis, some of which I refused to read initially because I felt that if I didn't acknowledge the horrific situation I found myself in it may go away.

As it turned out, much of the written word I received was very useful, with many articles providing knowledge that I had obviously missed during my own research and would prove useful when mapping out the road to my recovery. One such newspaper cutting was sent to me by my sister and was followed up by my daughter, who obtained further detailed information about the subject from a reliable source and expert.

When I read the article, I felt rather shocked and initially disappointed in the Spanish medical profession, which, up until that point, I had been very impressed with, especially the efficient and professional way I had been treated. Perhaps their failure to inform me of the possibility of any side effects that could arise from the removal of lymph nodes was because they believe that it is not necessary to raise the subject until an issue occurs. However, I would rather know all the facts related to the operation as I have always believed, ironically, that 'prevention is better than cure'!

A condition by the strange name of lymphoedema was now presenting itself as yet another hurdle I may encounter along the road to recovery and it seemed that, if I developed the condition, it would stay with me for many years to come. The story of a fellow breast-cancer sufferer with this condition was staring me in the face as I read the newspaper cutting and I was intrigued to find out what, how and why this had happened to her. The details outlined in the newspaper explained that sometimes, following breast cancer treatment and the removal of any lymph nodes (glands), a build-up of lymphatic fluid in the surface tissues in the armpit and surrounding tissue may occur. Once the lymph nodes are removed, they cannot be replaced so the lymphatic drainage routes are reduced. This condition does not happen to everyone who has had their lymph nodes removed and the degree to which an individual suffers will vary from person to person. Swelling, burning aching, throbbing, heaviness of limb and stiffness are some of the symptoms that occur following surgery or, in some cases, many years later.

The lady that was sharing her experience of lymphoedema had not been aware of the condition until the symptoms started to show themselves. It appeared that she had not been warned of the condition or, up until that point, had not been given any advice by her UK medical advisors as to how to deal with the condition. Fortunately, at the end of the article, there were contact details for the Lymphoedema Support Network (www.lymphoedema.org/lsn/index.html) and I was determined to find out as much information as I could from the appropriate source.

During the first few weeks, following the operation, I had

experienced some discomfort in my right arm, especially when trying to carry objects. Until I read the literature sent to me by the Lymphoedema Support Network, I had assumed that it was the after-effects of the surgery as it had been explained to me that it could take up to a year for the numbness to subside and for any sensation around the area where the lymph nodes had been removed to return. The heavy sensation was made worse by the numbness in the upper arm, armpit and left side, and I found myself relating to stroke victims!

The advice from the UK Lymphoedema Support Network and UK Breast Cancer Care (www.breastcancercare. org.uk) proved invaluable and thank goodness for these organizations who provide such a strong network of advisors. Details of their recommendations can be found in Part 2.

At this stage in my recovery, experiencing a few symptoms connected with this condition spurred me on to commence exercising more intensively, especially my upper body. Stretching became a regular part of my early morning routine as I endeavoured to accomplish the movement of raising my arms vertically above my head as far as it was possible and I involved Richard in regular massages of the affected area.

The soreness and pain of the horrific scarring proved to be an obstacle to overcome but I persevered and, slowly but surely, my movements became easier and complete elevation of my arm became possible without too much difficulty within six months.

I was pleased to pass on the knowledge about this associated condition of the lymph system to a fellow cancer sufferer, Jenny, that I had befriended and who had offered me a great deal of support and advice. She had never heard of it either and was very grateful for the details as, eighteen months after her lumpectomy, she developed acute lymphoedema and had to attend daily visits to the hospital for physiotherapy - demonstrating to us that the Spanish medical authorities seemed to offer very good treatment to those with lymphoedema who needed it. On a visit to the UK, I managed to track down a local National Health centre that specialized in care for Lymphoedema sufferers and they were able to give me advice on how to alleviate any swelling when travelling for long periods or flying long-haul.

However, I believe there is still a need for increased sharing of approaches and advice between the two countries on the subject of lymph node removal and making it available to all breast cancer sufferers.

It was now four months since I completed my chemotherapy and we were looking forward to a three-month holiday in the USA. This had been planned the year before and was to include a trip with my sister and her husband to Graceland and Nashville to celebrate my sister's sixtieth birthday. It also came at exactly the right time for a complete break away from any reminders of hospitals, medical jargon and the 'big C', or so I thought!

The flight to Florida, which was where we commenced our holiday, proved to be much more comfortable than I had expected. I had made sure I took on board the advice I had been given by the lymphoedema nurse and had spoken to an adviser at the clinic in Dorset about what precautions to take when flying or travelling for more than two hours in a confined space.

I was trussed up like a chicken with rather fetching

black support stockings that fitted right into my crutch. The reason for the stockings was to safeguard against deep-vein thrombosis which could be a side effect of the Tamoxifen (cancer drug) that I was now taking daily. My right arm was encased in a tight elasticated sleeve, which proved rather uncomfortable and gave the sensation that it was causing my arm to swell when, in fact, the opposite was true as the purpose of this compression garment is to encourage the lymph fluid to drain away from the affected arm. This elasticated sleeve provides a firm resistance against which the lymph vessels are squeezed by the muscles during activity, thus allowing the lymph fluid to move up the arm more effectively.

I had made sure I was wearing loose-fitting cotton trousers and top and, much to the annoyance of Richard and fellow passengers, I spent a great deal of the flight walking up and down and carrying out, in the toilet, strange exercises to stimulate my circulation. Drinking copious amounts of water also helped to prevent different parts of my body from swelling. An added bonus for me was that the jet lag proved to be minimal.

Ironically, it was poor Richard who had an uncomfortable start to the holiday as, within the first two weeks, he suffered a painful attack of gout! Having only ever been troubled with a very arthritic bunion, this condition proved most uncomfortable and the only explanation we can give is that he didn't drink much water on the flight and ate too much red meat (something he was not used to) on his arrival in the US. I am sure the previous stressful seven months had not helped his health either. Increasing his water consumption, elevating his feet and bandaging them with ice seemed to ease the problem.

It was during the second week, staying on the oceanside of the Gulf Coast, that we commenced our exercise regime. Consisting mainly of fast-walking and running, I decided I would also try to take advantage of the swimming pools and take a daily swim, which would also help the circulation in my right arm.

What a fabulous time we had in the coming weeks, visiting beautiful National Parks and beaches, swimming, running and walking every day, and visiting new parts of North-West Florida and discovering Northern central Florida as we travelled down to meet our daughter and her family further along the Gulf Coast. In every town we stayed, my restorative health protocol was never very far away and we would search out wonderful, well-stocked health food shops to replenish our supply of linseed/flax seed oil, supplements and organic foodstuffs.

The patience that Richard showed as he was subjected to ferrying me miles into inner cities to discover the latest health shop was overwhelming. The idiosyncrasies that I love about the USA, such as an easily available abundance of information on subjects such as cancer proved to be really informative and filled in a lot of gaps in my knowledge of holistic nutritional remedies. The ability to provide a variety of quality health products and give the consumer such choice at reasonable prices allowed me to stock up on items such as spirulina, wheat grass and barley grass.

As our holiday progressed I could feel my body getting stronger and stronger and I also noticed another change. My skin was becoming very shiny and it was no longer dry. My hair was also growing back, glossy, curly and strong. When I looked back over the last few years I had noticed that my skin and hair had been rather rough and noticeably dull. At the time I had thought these were symptoms that often accompany the menopause. I was always so conscious of not putting on too much weight and, rather than increase my calorie intake by including more oils in my diet, I would foolishly just slap on more skin moisturiser, not realizing that it was just as important to feed the skin from the inside.

I attributed the sudden change in my skin tone to the increase in the omega oils I was ingesting in the form of oily fish such as tinned sardines, fresh salmon, the linseed oil, olive oil, olives, nuts and seeds. Many articles I had read emphasized the importance of including the omega oils in one's daily diet as they contributed to the body's defence mechanism when fighting disease or helping to reduce the ageing process. These omegas were certainly making a marked difference to me, even if I was putting on weight.

The trip to the USA was proving to be a real tonic for restoring my body and mind to a more normal existence as I still heard, occasionally, a little voice of fear reminding me that the cancer could return. It seemed to enjoy wrestling with my overall determination to make a full recovery.

When our daughter and her family arrived for a two week break with us in Florida, they could see a marked improvement in my overall health and we had a wonderful time together, especially with our grandson, who was now walking and was so interested in everything around him. What joy I experienced when he entered our life and, at the most appropriate time, he gave me another reason to beat the disease that had temporarily attacked my body. During our daughter's time with us, we discovered that we were to be blessed with a second grandchild the following February.

We left Florida after a six week stay and flew to Tennessee to commence the second part of our holiday. This part of America was a new experience for us as we discovered the history of a country which claims to be so young. The origins of its diverse ancestors proved far more interesting than we had originally thought as we lost ourselves in local museums, National Parks and the folklore that abounds within the ancestry of the Native and African Americans.

Alongside our discoveries within this New World, we came across yet more health stores and a chance encounter with the owner of a health food store in Sevierville, the home town of the singer, Dolly Parton, was to be another turning point for me in my journey.

It was on our second visit to the Health store to stock up on my supply of flaxseed/linseed oil and digestive enzymes that I became engrossed in conversation with the assistant about a range of health products. She handed me a weekly newsletter written by an American M.D., Dr Sherry Rogers, who practised complementary remedies. This leaflet had several interesting articles, one of which caught my eye immediately (Total Wellness newsletter, September 2007, PO Box 3068, Syracuse, NY 13220)).

Back at our rented apartment, I read with interest the article entitled: 'Rescue from Cancer-causing Environmental Estrogens':

It has been known for a long time that prescribed estrogens may increase the breast cancer rate in some women, but scientists studying a higher rate of cancer in Long Island were surprised to discover that women in this area of America, with breast cancer, had higher levels of pesticides, such as DDT, in their breast compared with biopsies of normal breasts. These pesticides mimic the action of estrogen once they get into the body, and trigger cancer.

DDT is only the tip of the iceberg and we can discover, closer to home, how other products such as the cling-film we use to cover our food also contains these estrogen mimics. Babies' feeding bottles and the everyday plastic bottles that we buy our water in can leach nasty chemicals into our food and drink. Although the article, on first reading, appeared quite frightening, it went on to describe how we can 'rev up or supercharge our bodies' hormone detoxification pathways so that we can get rid of these xenoestrogens more efficiently. Rather than take up too much time in this chapter about the recommendations in the article, I have included the details in Part 2.

The excitement I felt at reading this new approach to help prevent the cancer returning reinforced my resolve to move forward with Dr Rogers' recommendations as soon as possible. The chance encounter with Bill, the owner of the store, and his assistant instigated a much longer-term professional relationship which proved very fruitful in providing me with objective advice on complementary theories, often tailored to suit my own personal needs.

For this, I will always be eternally thankful because the experience gave me even more resolve to continue with my preventative medicinal approach and convinced me even further of the power of positive-thinking and the responsibility we have to help ourselves.

We were nearing the end of our wonderful holiday and it was time to meet up with my sister and brother-in-law in Nashville for our exciting musical encounter with rock and roll and the King himself! No, he isn't alive but his music and personality certainly are, and what a musical-learning experience we all enjoyed. The beats of country, country and western, soul, blues and rock and roll music boomed night and day throughout Nashville and Memphis, transporting us to a musical sanctuary where no problems existed.

Well almost! I had continued my exercise regime throughout this period and managed to swim most days, determined to exercise my chest and arms and helping my lymph system as much as possible. However, throughout this period, I had constant nagging back-ache and, coincidently, my sister did too. As we compared notes, sitting in the sauna or swimming up and down in the pool, I tried to push any concerns I had to the back of my mind and enjoy the fun and laughter we were having in abundance!

On one such occasion, when we decided to go for an early morning swim, we were subjected to an extraordinary situation which could only happen in the USA and to my sister and me. We arrived at the empty, heated, indoor pool to commence our fifty or so lengths and, as usual, were not at a loss for subjects to talk about. Up and down we went, talking twenty to the dozen, Maggie on one side and me on the other, when all of a sudden a group of five people, three men and two women, arrived, fully clothed, at the edge of the pool.

They positioned themselves around one of the patio tables and I noticed the eldest man of the group was reading out loud from what looked like a Bible. We carried on swimming and I knew, without doubt, that Maggie was thinking the same thoughts as me: 'What on earth were they all doing, discussing religion in a stuffy, heated indoor swimming pool?!'

I stopped talking and carried on counting my tedious lengths and, to my utter amazement, three of the people entered the water from the shallow end, fully clothed. As I swam towards them on the return journey, I found it really difficult to prevent myself from laughing as I realized the bizarreness of the situation.

I dared not look at Maggie on the other side of the pool for fear of losing control, dissolving into fits of laughter and appearing really impolite. As the group moved towards the centre of the shallow end of the pool, we both realized that we couldn't carry on swimming as we were in the way and I felt it would appear very impolite. If we had jumped out of the water, we would have made too much noise, so we instinctively positioned ourselves in diagonal corners of the pool.

Very quickly, it became apparent that we were witnessing three baptisms, which involved head ducking the person under the water. The African-American Reverend said a prayer and the whole group followed up with 'Praised be the Lord.'

I watched the first person go under the water and, as she emerged, with her tight curly hair drenched and her black skin glistening from the water, once again I told myself this could only happen to Maggie and me, and only in the USA! Our husbands would never believe us, and this had all occurred before breakfast!

We patiently watched the other two baptisms and managed to suppress our jollity. Once the baptisms were over, the whole group hugged, dried themselves, thanked Maggie and me and went on their way as though it was the most normal procedure in the world to hijack a swimming pool at that time in the morning for three routine baptisms.

Without sounding disrespectful, we did have a great laugh about the set of circumstances we had found ourselves in. We were not laughing at the people or the actions they were taking but simply enjoying the humour of the moment. I have mentioned before how I love situational comedy. In fact, on reflection, we both agreed that it is one of America's great strengths, their lack of inhibitions and that nearly anything goes. I wish that we British would adopt a more liberal approach in our everyday lives and shed some of our 'stiff upper lip'.

Our three month holiday in America came to an end and I often look back with fondness on the wonderful times we had and really appreciate how therapeutic the whole experience was for both Richard and me. We returned to the UK for a short time and arrived back in Spain in time for my second six month check with my oncologist.

Chapter 19

Home and Dry?

SETTLING back into our life in Spain proved relatively easy and we were soon collecting our organic vegetables from the local organic farmer. Organic farming is very thin on the ground in Spain and we discovered this farmer through a recommendation from the local health food shop. Throughout the Costa del Sol, there is an abundance of smallholdings where the local farmers grow acres and acres of tomatoes the size of tennis balls, potatoes, peppers, aubergines, green beans, avocadoes, grapes, figs and citrus fruit. Unfortunately, there is a price to pay for ensuring that their harvests are so successful and this comes in the form of sprays which, whether or not they are deemed by the EU to be non-hazardous to health, are still substances that are not naturally formulated and may be responsible for some of the health problems we have in society today. Therefore, I always ensure I wash my salad foodstuffs and vegetables thoroughly, usually with vinegar or lemon juice added to a bowl of cold water.

The backache that had plagued me throughout the summer was still bothering me and I knew that I would have to mention it to the Oncologist at my forthcoming appointment. It was obvious that a series of tests would follow, which I was dreading, especially if it meant another MRI scan. The thought of entering that enclosed tube and being encased in the drum for what seemed like an eternity was etched on my mind. I never mentioned my fears to Richard or the children but, as the time went on and my backache didn't improve, I prayed constantly that it wasn't anything untoward. Knowing that bone cancer can occur as a secondary stage following breast cancer, I held onto the belief that my health regime would stand me in good stead for whatever the outcome may be. Anyway, my positive attitude believed that this road I was travelling had no room for any major holdups and I could see the light at the end of the tunnel getting closer and closer.

As I had predicted, my Oncologist sent me for a bone scan along with the usual chest x-ray and blood tests. The bone scan wasn't an MRI scan and proved to be a relatively straightforward procedure with dye being injected into my arm. Two hours following the administration of the initial injection, a scanner was used to scan my whole body. And this lasted approximately thirty to forty minutes and was not at all uncomfortable.

The young woman and man who administered the dye and carried out the bone scan could not have been more empathetic and seemed to sense my anxiety. When she took us back to the reception area and informed us to collect the results a few days later, I am sure I noticed her wink at me as if to say everything is ok. I hoped that this was not wishful thinking and vowed to try to block out any negative fears and busy myself until the appointment with the oncologist the following week.

When my appointment day arrived to collect my results, the anticipation as we sat in the waiting room presented itself in the form of déjà-vu and, although we didn't communicate very much, we both knew that the feelings we were experiencing were equally as difficult as the time I was originally diagnosed with cancer.

We were soon ushered into the consulting room. I handed the Doctor my results and, as we carried out the formalities of greeting one another, I was desperate to shout out, 'Tell me the verdict!'. However, I knew that the procedure for the first few minutes of the consultation would involve asking how I was and, therefore, we sat on the edge of our seats trying not to appear over-anxious! Finally, the oncologist presented the good news to us that the results were negative and there was no evidence of metastasis. I could have jumped up and hugged him. The relief was enormous and, as Richard described later, he felt as though he had won the lottery!

During that period, what surprised me was how both Richard and I were so visibly nervous and realised that all of the emotions and feelings of my previous diagnosis had come back to haunt us. When we both reflected on the situation, weeks later, we agreed that the nervous anxiety that we had experienced during the initial diagnosis and treatment had been buried whilst on holiday in the USA, and the process of having a bone scan resulted in these feelings manifesting themselves once more.

With the second check up out of the way and the all-clear being given, I was determined to settle back and enjoy the Spanish sunshine and the company of our dear friends before our return to the UK in November. My mother joined us for a month and our children were constantly on the 'phone or using Skype to communicate via the computer, which proved extremely useful as we were missing our little grandson desperately.

It was during the many chats that we had with our daughter that it became apparent that we would be spending longer periods in the UK. The prospect of having another grandchild was also another prompt for us in rethinking our lives. This was a great relief to Paula who never expressed openly her desire for us to return to the UK on a more permanent basis, until one day in an emotional outburst she declared that she wished we were just down the road.

This was not surprising when you consider what we had experienced over the past twelve months as a family and realising that we could make ourselves useful helping out with the grandchildren when our daughter returned to work, we made preparations to stay for longer periods in the UK. When one experiences one's own mortality, you soon realise that every moment spent with your loved ones is so valuable.

The past twelve years in Spain had been a great experience and I can honestly say, apart from the usual ups and downs that happen when living in a foreign country, our time was one of the happiest periods of our life. We have met some very good people who have all proved to be priceless friends, especially during my journey to recovery.

The decision to stay in Spain during my treatment and not return to the bosom of my family proved for me to be the right one as the medical profession, climate and support group of friends all, I believe, contributed a great deal to the restoration of my health. I know that, generally, my immediate family would have preferred me to have returned to England so that they could have helped in my care but, overall, everything worked out for the best. I certainly had not wanted to be faced with watching the heartache and worry that my illness was causing my mother, siblings and close family whilst in my recovery period. It was traumatic enough being aware of the sadness that my children and husband were suffering.

One of the lessons I have learnt is that the cancer journey involves the patient, for a period of time, becoming very focused on themselves and their own health and well being. I realised early on that if you do not devote positive time and energy to ridding your body of the cancer then you cannot expect to return to full health.

It didn't take us long to sell our apartment and we managed to rent another in an area close to the sea, whilst we decided what we would do, longer term, regarding the property market. There was no urgency to find a new home as my decision to have reconstructive surgery, using a relatively new pioneering technique, would certainly take up some of the next year of our life and would mean renting accommodation close to the hospital in Norwich.

Packing up boxes once more became part of our life for the next few weeks. However, we were soon on our way to the UK to stay with our daughter before spending a family Christmas in Qatar with our son.

Chapter 20

Chicken Fillets

THE first time I tried on my bathing costume during the first few days of our Floridian holiday, I had not taken too much notice of my out-of-proportion figure with its flat sunken chest and thick thighs. As I wrapped myself in a sarong and convinced myself that I looked just fine and that nobody, in a land overflowing with cosmetically-enhanced ladies, would be looking at me! I was right! No one around the pool appeared to be noticing me too much.

I managed to slip into the water whilst it was relatively empty and positioned my towel and clothes where they would be easily accessible so that when I heaved myself up out of the water, I could cover myself up discretely, away from prying eyes. All was going well until a handsome family appeared and situated themselves next to my sun bed and clothes. To make matters worse, the wife had an 'awesome' figure and was wearing a stylish bikini. Whilst swimming, I worked on a strategy of how I could climb out of the pool without having to show the front of my torso! Impossible! At the end of my swim, I took a deep breath, heaved myself out of the shallow end and walked around to my clothes. Not even stopping to dry myself, I embarrassingly gathered up my belongings and walked briskly back to the apartment.

Up until that point in my recovery, I had resisted the temptation to search out mastectomy bras and prostheses. This was partly because I could not be bothered with the inconvenience of wearing them every day and partly because I had convinced myself that I didn't need them as I wasn't a vain lady and such things would not bother me! How wrong I was and it was at that moment, during that first swim in Florida, that I realized I was not going to get through my vacation without investigating the possibility of some false boobs!

Reconstruction had been discussed several times between Richard and myself and Richard had even gone as far as investigating different options available for me. However, I had always left the subject very much up in the air not wanting to consider any more surgery for the foreseeable future and Richard had never put any pressure on me to follow through with a reconstruction operation, simply saying that, as long as I was well, that was all that mattered.

On returning to the apartment that day, I expressed to him how I was feeling and that, suddenly, it wasn't ok for me to be breastless. After a really fruitful discussion, we came to the conclusion that we would visit the local shopping mall and search out a mastectomy bra and swim suit. America could be a good place to receive the type of guidance I would need on what type of products were available for women in my situation.

The first store we entered was an upmarket swimwear shop with beautiful designer bathing costumes and beach wear. Once I had explained my requirements, the sales assistant couldn't do enough to help me and it was great fun rummaging through the racks of swim suits deciding

152

which were interchangeable for use with the prosthesis. As there was so much choice I soon found one that made me look more womanly and the assistant showed me how to insert the jelly-like 'chicken fillets'. Although grateful that I had found this shop, which would solve my breastless problem, as with my wig, I still couldn't say I ever became very fond of the whole process of dressing up in my false 'boobs'.

Next stop would be to find a shop that supplied mastectomy bras that would house my false fillets when I was not swimming. Close by was a large shopping mall and, because the swimwear shop had stocked mastectomy swimsuits, we naively thought that the women's attractive underwear shop, that had caught our eye, would provide us with just what we were looking for. It was not to be! Discovering from a member of staff that they didn't have a mastectomy bra section, we asked whether she knew where there was a shop which would supply them.

By this time we were standing at the till and all of a sudden, at the top of her voice, in front of all of the customers, the assistant let out, in her loud American drawl, a request to her colleague on the other side of the shop: ' do you know where this lady can buy mastectomy bras from?' Well I don't know who was more embarrassed, Richard, because he was a man in a lady's underwear shop looking for mastectomy bras, or me because I was the customer they were making the fuss about! A few suggestions were shouted back and we made a hasty red-faced retreat. Stepping out into the blazing Floridian sun we both saw the funny side of it and agreed once again that such a humorous situation could only happen in the USA.

Failing to come up with any suitable mastectomy bras and wanting to use the same chicken fillets that I had bought for my swimsuit, it was decided to buy an ordinary sports bra which was lined and try to replicate the type of opening made in the swimsuit. This would house my new prosthesis and it worked a treat. Fully equipped with my new bras and swim suit I was ready to continue my beach holiday, less self-conscious for both Richard and myself.

It was inevitable that this process of organising my new underwear would bring to the surface the question of reconstruction and, during this period, we took the opportunity to mull over the alternatives and discuss when and where I could have the operation. The thought of spending the rest of my life ensuring my spongy implants were in-situ and trailing around underwear shops looking for suitable bras made the thought of yet more surgery bearable.

One other key figure that was very important in this whole debate was Richard. Knowing him as I do, I knew that the majority of the time he really did not care that his wife had no breasts. However, it would be very unfair to suggest that he is different from other men and, although he never said, I knew he was bothered about the effect it may have longer term on our physical relationship.

Until you have no breasts - not small ones - I really mean no breasts, you do not realise the role they play in your life. As well as the most obvious functions such as breast-feeding, etc, it is surprising how cold you feel, how clothes hang differently and how your balance is affected.

Therefore, the research began in earnest, looking at breast reconstruction techniques available and, as I didn't favour silicone or saline implants, I was interested to discover what alternative materials were available to build my new breasts.

CHAPTER 21

'THE BOUDICA WITHIN'

IN the weeks following my diagnosis, I had very kindly been bombarded with articles, newspaper cuttings and helpful advice about breast cancer or examples of individuals who had experience of the disease. At the time a lot of the information was put safely to one side due to my feeling that I was experiencing 'information overload'.

Remembering a comment made some years earlier by the husband of one of our staff, who unfortunately succumbed to ovarian cancer and had taken part in the early trails of Tamoxifen, that a little knowledge is a dangerous thing, I attempted to classify in order of priority what I needed to read and action without further adding to the initial state of panic I had found myself in. The nearest example I am able to give to compare with the inner dread I felt trying to digest the quantities of literature available, plus the research Richard and I were carrying out on the subject of cancer, was when you are confronted with the first stages of revision when sitting exams! 'Where do I begin?'

As time went on and I became more in control of my own healing protocol I was able to commence reading, at my leisure, the material that I had originally put to one side.

One day, when sorting through my bedside drawer, I found a two-page spread from a daily tabloid which had been given to me by a well-read friend. Initially the article had filled me with an ignorant horror as I had skimmed the pages, discovering examples of women who had received breast reconstruction using their own tissue. I thought the procedure sounded like something out of a Frankenstein film script and stuffed it back in the drawer. When I eventually reread the article, I soon realised that ignorance is not bliss, and how wrong I had been to formulate such a hasty first impression.

That morning, as I lay in bed with Richard, devouring the written information with a completely different attitude, staring me in the face was an array of very brave and beautiful women who had all agreed to the reconstruction of their breasts using a new pioneering technique, which involved transplanting their own tissue.

Having Richard peering over my shoulder, absorbing the information, helped a great deal as he was able to add to my thoughts with his usual intelligent, constructive, objective viewpoints. By this time, I had been reduced to a blubbering mess due to a wave of empathy that had swept over me as I read their stories. I knew just how they had felt, following the surgery to remove their cancers.

At the end of the article were the details of the Surgeon who had been trained by the original American pioneer of the procedure. It was evident that this highly-trained lady had successfully facilitated the restructuring not only of these women's breasts but, also, of their lives. I noted with interest that a book had been written with examples of some of the women, sharing their experiences of this type of surgery. I definitely wanted a copy and it was at this moment that my relationship with 'The Boudica Within' was formed.

As I was busy trying to implement the immune-building protocol designed for me by my complementary therapist, Richard took it upon himself to research into this relatively new technique for breast reconstruction and to find out more about the surgeons available world-wide who had the expertise to implement the procedure. As I had only just finished my chemotherapy and had still not quite come to terms with the idea of having breast reconstruction, I was very grateful that Richard was carrying out the initial fact-finding mission.

He provided me with information on the traditional breast reconstruction techniques so that I could compare the risks and benefits with the new type of surgery. However, the thought of inserting a foreign object into my body such as a silicone or a saline sac, as well as replacing it every ten to fifteen years, especially since the removal of my cancer lump and total breast tissue, made me feel instinctively very uncomfortable.

The overall research exposed many interesting facts, some of which are available in the second part of Part 2. One such piece of information described one of the world's leading breast reconstruction surgeons in this type of procedure, an American surgeon, Dr Bob Allen (http://www.diepflap.com/index.html), who had pioneered the revolutionary technique and was invited to the UK in 2005 to pass on his expertise to surgeons at the Norfolk and Norwich University Hospital. Coincidentally, the invitation had come from consultant plastic surgeon, Elaine Sassoon (http://www.elainesassoon.com/), whom we had read about in the tabloid article.

In August of that year, Dr Allen 'had carried out for the first time in Britain a ground-breaking variation of the pioneering operation, reconstructing a female breast using

fatty tissue from the patient rather than muscle or implants.'
He also went on to pass on his expertise to surgeons in
the region including, obviously, Ms Sassoon. Further
research showed that there were several variations of the
technique and each operation used a technique that was
suitable for the individuals' body shape. Although similar
methods of restructuring have been around for many years,
the important difference about this technique was that,
wherever possible, removal of the patient's muscle was
avoided, ensuring that long-term recovery would be more
comfortable.

The Norfolk and Norwich University Hospital was not
the only hospital to offer the technique and we discovered
that there were expert surgeons in Barcelona and at St
Thomas's, London. However, we decided to look, initially,
at two options: we would visit a cosmetic breast specialist
in Malaga, recommended to us by the surgeon who had
carried out my bi-lateral mastectomy, and write to and visit
the Norfolk and Norwich Specialist and then compare our
findings. I knew that any decision made would rest crucially
on my 'gut' instinct as to who I would feel most comfortable
with and what procedure was right for me.

The appointment in Malaga was not a huge success
and it had got off to a bad start when we entered a rather
dreary looking office in the older part of the City, which
did nothing to build confidence in a new patient awaiting
breast reconstruction advice. After an incredibly long wait,
watching various women, some of whom had plasters and
eye patches on their faces, going in and out of a small office,
we were called into the same office to see the surgeon.

Sitting down, I remember thinking that I was now
entering the world of plastic surgery, a world that had never

really interested me until now. It was a difficult and stilted conversation conducted totally in Spanish as the consultant appeared to have little or no English. After her initial examination of my chest and clarifying what my original bust size had been, we sat down to discuss the options available to me. Her demeanour was one of disinterest especially when we asked her if she could provide other options to the traditional breast reconstruction she had described.

Reemphasising that she only offered silicone or saline implants, using the expander technique, through Richard's superb translation skills, I thanked her for her help and said I would think about it, knowing full well that her strange manner had done nothing to endear me to her as my prospective breast reconstruction surgeon.

To date, I had always formed cordial if not affectionate relationships with the medical profession that treated me and I knew it was crucial to the success of my treatment to feel relaxed when interacting with these experts. The throughput of clients we saw during our time in the waiting room led me to believe that the whole experience of this particular clinic would be the stereotypical plastic surgery approach, 'wheel them in and wheel them out'.

Only four months after being told I had cancer, my nerves were still extremely raw and I was convinced I would remain in this fragile and shaky state for ever. Although at no time during my treatment and recovery did I want to be treated with kid gloves, I did not respond well to individuals who displayed no empathy at all for my plight.

Some women who lose their breasts understandably feel as though they have lost their femininity and are no longer sexually desirable to the opposite sex. I can completely understand these emotions. However, for me there was only one man that I wanted to sexually desire me and that was my husband. At no time did I feel less of a woman because of the demise of my breasts and my sex life remained as it always had, extremely fulfilling.

Vanity was not a problem, either, as I knew I was no Sophia Lauren and I had always tried to make the best of my assets and hide my bodily deficiencies. Therefore, what was driving me down the path of breast reconstruction? Although disappointed and a little disillusioned with the first breast reconstruction consultation, the fact-finding continued and arrangements were made to see the Norfolk and Norwich Cosmetic Specialist in April when we returned to the UK for Richard to run the London Marathon in aid of Breast Cancer.

Our journey to Norwich proved interesting in more ways than one. Encountering a delightful city which would become very familiar to us over the coming year, discovering an amazing university hospital, which, on first viewing gave the impression of a state of the art medical city, which housed, I later discovered, amazingly dedicated and well-trained medical staff and, last but not least, a very stylish, interesting, if slightly eccentric, female surgeon.

Our first impression of this lady was that she behaved in a very professional business-like manner and she obviously did not suffer fools gladly. Although I can honestly say I did not instantly warm to her at the start of the first meeting, instinctively I felt that the confidence she demonstrated in her subject was all that mattered.

Her lack of eye contact when you talked to her was not to be mistaken for disinterest in her clients and I experienced on many occasions her piercing, foreign-looking eyes, weighing me up and down. Her insistence on directing all of her questions and the passing on of information directly to me and at times ignoring Richard completely proved disconcerting, especially as Richard and I always discussed everything. This behaviour, I concluded, was due to the surgeon ensuring that the female requesting the new breasts was the only one making the final decision on the reconstruction procedure with no influence from outside sources.

Once all of my details had been given to Ms Sassoon and she had finished her examination of me, she gave us information about the type of operations available and which one would be suitable for me. Now that I had got over my original horror of the thought of transplanting tissue from one part of the body to another, I listened in earnest to the various options. She was recommending the surgery that used the tummy tissue, although, looking down at my abdomen, I didn't see how there was enough tissue to create two decent size breasts.

Here is a simple description of the very complicated procedure:

'Approximately eight years previously, a new procedure in the restructuring of breasts commenced and was named by Dr Bob Allen as the 'Perforator Flap Technique'. It was called thus because the surgeon takes a flap of 'tissue which includes the skin and fat with one single artery and vein from the abdomen or the buttocks and sews them to the mastectomy site. The operations are delicate and involve complex microsurgery (the use of small needles and suture to sew blood vessels together using an operating microscope).

The small blood vessels that enter the fat are reconnected to recipient blood vessels beneath the arm or on the chest. This restores blood circulation through the tissue and allows it to heal into place in its new position. When the flap is getting a good blood supply, tucking and pleating the tissue commences to fashion the new breast, moulding the transferred tissue to create a new one similar to the other one.

The advantage to the patient is that no muscle is taken with the flap, only skin and fat, thereby minimising the risk of weakness and hernia of the abdominal wall and a mesh is not needed. There is usually enough tissue to build a breast without the use of an implant, so the result should be permanent. The abdomen is tightened as in a "tummy tuck" or the buttock is sewn as in a "buttock lift".

It is major surgery lasting from five to eight hours and requiring about six days in hospital. Although the failure rate is now quite low, the procedure requires lengthy surgery and a long recovery period.

Every breast and flap is different, so precisely what has to be carried out will vary between patients. When the surgeon is happy with the shape, they close up with under-the-skin stitches, which give the best cosmetic result.

Patients are monitored every half hour over the first 48 hours to check that the new breast has a good blood supply. If the breast goes cold or white, one of the joined vessels is blocked. This could mean emergency surgery to repair the problem. Patients stay in hospital for a week and will initially be on a high protein diet. The complete recovery period is usually four to six weeks.'

(http://www.elainesassoon.com/Download%20files/ BREAST%20RECONSTRUCTION.doc)

Armed with the details that had been given to us by Ms Sassoon at the first consultation in Norwich and the written information that Richard had gleaned from the Internet, we felt that it was just a matter of digesting the facts and making a decision. Ms Sassoon had suggested waiting until September for the operation in order to give my body more time to recover from the chemotherapy. As we were going on holiday to Florida, this seemed to be a sensible decision.

Travelling back by train to where our daughter lived on the UK south coast, my mind was full of all kinds of concerns and worries and I tried to distract myself with the book I had just bought, which had been written by Elaine Sassoon, detailing examples of her previous breast reconstruction patients. As I sat on Norwich station waiting for the train, I flicked through the pages of the book.

As Ms Sassoon explains in the introduction to her book, 'Boudica' means 'Bringer of Victory'. 'The Boudica Within' was an apt title for the book as it contained sensitive stories of women who have taken the extraordinary journey through breast cancer and their experiences of breast reconstruction.

The book was a tribute to Ms Sassoon's patients who, over the past ten years, had impressed her with their 'fortitude, resilience and sense of humour.' She had observed many times how they had changed from victims to extraordinary women who discovered inner strengths they never knew they possessed. What was so unusual about the concept of the book was the photography that surrounded each case study. Tastefully and sensually photographed were a group of amazing women, proudly displaying their newly-constructed breasts. These were real women, some young, some older, some whose reconstruction operations had been very difficult for Ms Sassoon and others who still displayed immature red scars.

She was not interested in air-bushing out their imperfections or only selecting the best results and, yet, what springs from the pages of the book are beautiful photographs of attractive women delighted with their newly-formed bodies. The three wonderful locations for the shoots, a farm, a beautiful garden and a Norfolk beach, all added to the atmosphere of what the book was trying to portray.

As I turned the pages, with tears streaming down my face and in absolute awe of these very brave Boudicas, I came to the conclusion there was a strong possibility I would be joining them in the decision to have this type of breast reconstruction.

With Richard successfully completing the London Marathon, we returned to Spain and I continued with my complementary immune-building protocol. Over the next two months, we familiarised ourselves with the terminology of the new breast reconstruction procedures and Richard became very proficient in quoting the abbreviations of the various breast 'perforator flap' techniques: D.I.E.P., I.G.A.P., S.G.A.P. etc. We also had more of an understanding of when a traditional implant was used or a combination of procedures and of the breast cosmetic surgery services available. This made a welcome relief from talking about breast cancer.

Many discussions later, it was decided that we would contact Elaine Sassoon to inform her that I was happy - well not exactly happy, rather terrified actually - to go ahead with the operation. However, mulling over the option of having the tissue removed from my abdomen, I decided that I would rather use my bottom to formulate the new breasts. The main reason being that where I had lost weight during my chemotherapy, it didn't look to me as though there was enough fat available to provide me with two decent size new breasts. My buttocks were far more sizeable!

Although I wasn't interested in acquiring a chest the size of Jordan, I certainly did not want to go through all of the pain and discomfort of the DIEP operation and not have anything worthwhile to show for it! We e-mailed Ms Sassoon's secretary and confirmed the appointment in June, agreed a date for mid-September for the operation and explained that I had changed my mind and now wanted two IGAP operations. Two operations would be required on two separate dates, at least three months apart due to the fact that the type of surgery involved in the IGAP procedure required the surgeons to only work on one side of the body at a time.

Just before we flew to Florida, we made our second trip to see Ms Sassoon in Norwich to finalise the arrangements for the operation and for her to carry out another assessment of me. Psychologically, I was prepared for my breast reconstruction operation but, it seems, my body was not. I had taken with me to the appointment my latest blood test results from my first six-monthly check up with the oncologist, as I thought they would be of interest in determining how fit my body was for the operation. They did prove useful as I think they helped Elaine in determining that I really was not yet strong enough to have such major surgery.

Naturally, I was very disappointed that she wanted to cancel the operation until January as I just wanted it out of the way and to get on with my life. Richard tried to console me by stressing that it was really important that I was strong and healthy when undergoing such an operation and, slowly, I got used to the idea of the postponement.

Due, I am sure, to the IGAP operation seeming to be a far more complicated procedure as both buttocks would be involved, Elaine rather reluctantly agreed to carry out the rebuilding of my breasts using this technique. I was introduced to a fellow surgeon who would work with her in the theatre.

We agreed another appointment for September and Ms Sassoon wished me well and told me to exercise and get as strong as I could in preparation for the surgery in January.

The American holiday was to be a great opportunity to heed her advice and the following two months proved to be just what the Doctor had ordered! Swimming, walking and running ensured that I continued to improve my circulation in my right arm and strengthen my limbs, especially in the places that mattered for the forthcoming operation such as the upper body. It was essential that I had a healthy supply of blood vessels available in the chest area to ensure that any transfer of tissue would be successful in establishing itself in its new home.

Although, during this time, I didn't dwell too much on my decision to have breast reconstruction, our time spent in America didn't prove completely trouble free from the subject matter. We received an e-mail from Ms Sassoon's secretary informing us that our private medical insurance company were refusing to cover all of the costs of the surgeon's fees because they were deemed too high and querying why there was a need for two surgeons.

After many transatlantic 'phone calls and frantic discussions with other surgeons whom we had tracked down that were qualified to perform the operation about their charges, we managed to convince the insurance company that the quote given to us by Ms Sassoon's team for the required surgery was competitively priced. The surgery is available on the National Health Service in Norfolk but because I was resident in Spain I would only qualify if I returned to the UK for six months prior to the operation.

Fortunately, we had taken out private medical insurance when we moved to Spain, twelve years previously, and, to date, we had never had any problems with the insurance company. Indeed, after this blip in the approval process for the breast reconstruction, all of our claims were processed efficiently.

September soon arrived and I was very relieved when Ms Sassoon finally agreed to carry out the surgery. A date was finalised for the beginning of January 2009.

CHAPTER 22

FIGHTING INFECTIONS

AS is usually the case in my life, the period between September and January was, fortunately, taken up with a great deal of activity so I did not have too much time to dwell on my impending operation. We returned to Spain for my six-monthly check and settled into our life in Spain with my mother joining us for the month of October.

Completely out of the blue, we were contacted by a friend who was searching for a three-bedroom apartment and he wanted to know if our apartment was for sale! As Richard always says: 'Everything has a price'. Although we were not looking to sell, having only been in our new home a year, the request came coincidentally, at a time when, due to the life-changing upheaval we had experienced over the past months, I was starting to have doubts about whether I wanted to remain in Spain, away from my grandson and family.

I had not broached the subject of returning to the UK with Richard as I knew the thought of giving up our wonderful Mediterranean lifestyle for the cold dark winter days ahead would not appeal to him at all. However, the pull of wanting to make the most of every moment with our grandchildren and share in their lives was proving too strong.

Fate had stepped in and made the decision for us and, to the delight of our daughter and son-in-law, the apartment was sold and, with Richard admitting that he felt the same as I did about missing our family, we returned to the UK in December. We knew the year ahead would be filled with hospital appointments and operations, culminating in a disjointed way of life, so we didn't make any immediate plans as to where we were going to live. When we weren't in Norwich, we would live with our daughter and son-in-law.

When we arrived in the UK, the November weather in the South of England didn't seem too bad and, as we had left behind snow on the mountains of Southern Spain, we were quite glad to feel the cosiness of an English home. This was not for long, though, as we had all booked flights to spend Christmas in Qatar with our son and had agreed to fly out earlier to help him prepare for the Christmas festivities. This was an exciting time as we would all be together to share in our grandson's second Christmas experience and the weather would be hot!

Whilst in Qatar, I developed a bladder infection and my son whisked me off to the nearby state of the art medical clinic for treatment. Following a serious of tests, it was discovered that I had a vaginal infection caused through the bacteria streptococcus, which was travelling, understandably, into my urine. Over the past few weeks, I had not felt as well as I had done in America and was concerned that my immune system was failing me.

My last blood-test had shown that the white blood count was still lower than it should be and the Oncologist had pointed this out, saying, in broken English, that the body was still struggling to recover from the chemotherapy treatment. So I was aware that I would be prone to still more infections. The antibiotics that I was given to clear up my bacterial infection seemed to do the trick and I was able to continue with my holiday without any more interference from my health issues.

This vaginal problem had flared up a couple of times before and my gynaecologist had explained, simplistically, that this was the internal bacteria and fungi that reside in the vagina becoming out of balance, probably due to my age.

Therefore, I was not unduly worried, just fed up with continually feeling below par. I have mentioned before that, although I am not comfortable with becoming too self-indulgent when I am ill and always try to remain upbeat, it was during this period that I became increasingly frustrated with the slow recovery that my body was making and the fact that there always seemed something wrong with me.

My breast reconstruction surgeon had insisted that I stop all vitamin supplements three months before my operation as, apparently, any that may have the effect of thinning the blood could have a detrimental effect on me during the operation. Being extremely competent in her profession as a surgeon and the fact that there would be the need to ensure that my blood vessels fused together successfully, she wasn't going to take any chances with my suffering what the medical profession terms 'a bleed'.

However, by suddenly not receiving the necessary additional nutrients from my complementary health protocol, my body's immune system may have been impaired and, therefore, I was more open to picking up infections. My common sense told me that this could not be helped and, if I was to successfully acquire new breasts, then a compromise needed to be made and I would just have to put up with not feeling one hundred per cent fit and well.

Thank goodness that I had the Christmas holiday to distract me and I was determined to make the most of this wonderful experience with my adorable family. I pushed to the back of my mind the thought that my body still may not be ready for my breast reconstruction operation in January.

Our son was the perfect host and we all agreed that we would do it again soon, as this family holiday had proved such a huge success.

Back in the UK, the 2009 New Year celebrations came and went and, during the days leading up to the operation, I went down with a very bad cough and cold. The accommodation in Norwich had been booked for six weeks and, with our cases packed, we headed east towards the Norfolk coast, fingers and toes crossed that the chest infection, which had now developed, would clear up by the time Ms Sassoon carried out her pre-operative assessment.

It took a couple of days to settle into the little two-bedroom cottage we had rented, just enough time to unpack, stock up on foodstuffs and familiarise ourselves with our new surroundings before 'D' day, or should I say 'B' day! I had been warned that I would not be able to do very much for the first few weeks following my operation and, as Richard would be backwards and forwards to the hospital, I wanted to make sure that our home life would be as organised as possible for when I came out. Richard would be under enough pressure being a full-time carer without having to think initially about too many domestic duties.

The pre-operative assessment day arrived and, as we approached the Norfolk and Norwich University Hospital for the first time, my mouth dropped open at the site of the campus-like buildings which were so vast. Once inside, the interconnected buildings ran like a maze west to east and north to south and gave the impression of a space-age bustling citadel. Eventually we located the area of the hospital which accommodated the plastic surgery department and the private wing.

Once we had found the appropriate ward, the nursing sister registered my details and the usual series of tests were carried out by very pleasant staff on my heart, blood and blood pressure. I met with the anaesthetist who, after examining me, became aware that I had a chest infection. Despite my attempts to conceal the sore throat and croaky voice there was no disguising the fact that this chest infection was not going away. I questioned him about whether the operation would still go ahead if I was not a hundred percent and, to my relief, he said it probably would.

We managed to grab a bowl of soup for lunch and then met up with the nurse who would take me to the MRI scanner clinic where I had an appointment. Having previously experienced two MRI scans for a knee injury I had contracted, I was not looking forward to forty minutes lying on my back, encased in a claustrophobic metal drum and unable to move.

It was important for the surgeons to have clear images of where the appropriate blood vessels were in my tummy and chest area and this was the reason for the lengthy scan. A dye would be injected into me during the time I was being x-rayed. Unfortunately, it took about half an hour, several attempts and the assistance of a doctor before finally a needle was successfully attached to my hand. The nursing staff had given up on my left arm as my veins were proving difficult to penetrate. One of the nurses told me that apparently this can sometimes happen because the veins collapse as a result of the chemotherapy and they don't always recover. It was not possible to use the right arm due to the risk of infection. At no time was I to be given any injections, blood taken or my blood pressure checked in my right arm, which was pre-disposed to lymphoedema (this is the arm from where my lymph nodes had been removed).

Eyes tightly shut, I entered the MRI scanner with trepidation, especially when the nurse said it would be about an hour before I was released from my metal tomb. She could sense I was nervous and reassured me by saying that she would play some relaxing music. Chatting away to myself in my head I decided that I would take the opportunity to relax and sleep a little in preparation for my operation the following day. I also prayed I wouldn't cough.

My bad throat, which still refused to go away, occasionally without warning, provoked an attack of coughing and, if this occurred while I was being photographed, the whole x-ray would be ruined. I focused intently on the music and the instructions that came over the loud speaker from an unknown voice informing me of when I should breathe deeply or hold my breath. After what seemed like an eternity the voice told me that it would only be another five minutes and then I would be able to escape. Thank goodness, because I had lost count of how many times the one classical piece of music had been played! It was the longest five minutes of my life and I am, to this day, sure those final five minutes turned into about twenty.

Eventually, I was pulled out of the tunnel and, as I had not opened my eyes the whole time I was in there, it took a while to get me back on my feet and for my eyes to adjust to the light. Still shaking when I was reunited with Richard, I knew that I had to get a grip and pull myself together as I couldn't go down to theatre the following day so tense. Richard beamed a smile at me and, looking at his watch, informed me that I had been gone two hours. I wasn't surprised at the timescale and reckoned I had been in the scanner about ninety minutes.

By late afternoon my bed was ready for me and I was relieved to hear that the operation was to be carried out the following morning at 8.00 a.m. At least I wouldn't be hanging around without any breakfast and there would not be much time for me to become too nervous. The private room I had been given was very comfortable but cold and, at the time of my arrival, it housed an electrician who was busy up a ladder with his head in the loft area of the false ceiling. This was a welcome distraction from what lay ahead and Richard made polite conversation with him, finding out that he was investigating an air-conditioning problem.

Just as I was enjoying a nice cup of tea, a nurse suddenly appeared, asking me if I would like to order some dinner for that evening. Looking at my watch, I couldn't believe it was dinner time already and I was relieved that they hadn't forgotten me. I didn't relish the thought of being kept awake all night by a rumbling tummy and, as if by magic, a plate of fish, jacket potato and peas soon arrived and, with the electrician still up the ladder, I attempted to devour my dinner.

All of a sudden, the door flew open and there stood my surgeon, as always very glamorously dressed. Looking tired, she enquired of the man up the ladder in the middle of the room what he was up to, as well as emphasising that it was far too cold in the room. Apparently, it was essential that I was kept very warm, which would ensure that my blood vessels were fully dilated in preparation for my operation the following morning. She requested that I stand up so she could examine me and I reluctantly pushed my dinner away, knowing full well that when I eventually was able to eat it, it would be even colder than when it had first arrived.

It was time for Ms Sassoon to draw on my body exactly where the new breasts would be located and she asked me to remove my dressing gown and pyjamas. The electrician obviously heard this request because he sprinted back down the ladder, stating that he could come back later. I was relieved that I didn't have to bare my scar-ridden, naked body to a complete stranger. It was bad enough exposing it to the surgeon.

As the electrician made a speedy exit from the room, I made some quip about the current situation being like something out of a comedy script.

Using her black marker pen, Ms Sassoon drew the necessary markings on my chest area and enquired as to whether I had been down to x-ray for the ultrasound scan that had been scheduled for me at five o'clock. This was news to me and, rather irritated, she instructed me to get dressed and she would take me herself as the radiographer would be waiting for us.

She disappeared to find a heater for my room and I agreed with Richard that he should go back to the cottage. He had also had a long day with a lot of waiting around and there was no telling how long this other x-ray would take. He wished me luck and we embraced lovingly just as the surgeon came back with a heater. She gave Richard details of when to telephone and visit the following day and informed me that I would be moving to a warmer room later that evening.

We then set off on a route march to the other side of the hospital to complete my ultrasound scan. This was deemed necessary because the period I had earlier spent in the MRI scanner had proved a total waste of time with only poor images being recorded. This can happen if a patient moves at the wrong moment. The one good thing about all of the tests I endured that day was that the time went quickly and I kept thinking this time tomorrow it will all be over. Although I am not an advocate of wishing one's life away, especially after my recent life-changing experience, in certain circumstances it works and makes the situation that you are not looking forward to almost bearable.

Returning to my hospital room, after a reprimand from my surgeon about the state of my croaky voice and her emphasising once more how important it was that I was free of all viruses due to the high risk of pneumonia following the operation, I never felt so alone in all my life. The comment that she was not happy about operating on me in my condition only added to the despondency I was feeling. I knew she was right and all of the gargling and inhaling with Olbas Oil over the past few days had done nothing to improve my chest and I just prayed that she wouldn't change her mind about carrying out the operation the next day.

My prayers were answered by her colleague, who would be assisting in the rebuilding of my new chest. A rather large, jolly-faced man, and another Richard, he appeared that evening at the end of a very long day for him and me, to offer support and, more importantly, to answer any questions I might have. Well, never at a loss for words or questions, I can honestly say I don't remember what I asked him that night as he sat on my bed, I just know he was a great comfort and his confidence gave me the affirmation that I was doing the right thing by going through with this type of operation.

He also quietly reassured me, as the anaesthetist had done earlier that day, that it was highly likely the operation would go ahead. I was beginning to understand the dynamics of this particular plastic surgery team, how all of the players were different, how each brought a unique personality and phenomenal medical skills, which culminated in such a high success rate when carrying out what is known as the perforated flap technique. My confidence was increasing the more I interacted with the hospital staff and, as Surgeon Richard bid me goodnight and promised to pop in at seven the next morning to see how I was, I felt comfortable that my life on the operating table would be in very good hands.

Feeling a lot better by the time he had left, I was determined to get an early night as I knew I would be awoken early by the hospital routine. I was moved to what proved to be a stiflingly hot room, which I knew I would have to grin and bear for Elaine Sassoon's sake, if not my own, and settled myself down to sleep. It was a fitful night's sleep and I dozed on and off until about five-thirty when I took myself into the bathroom for a shower and a final attempt at coughing up the mountains of phlegm that seemed to collect every night in the back of my throat. At this stage I wasn't too nervous. However, I did not feel one hundred per cent well and the ulcers that had plagued me on and off over the year had returned with a vengeance.

The night staff had informed me that I would be going down to theatre at about seven-thirty and, as I wouldn't be having any breakfast, I decided to investigate the ward I was in and familiarise myself with my surroundings. It was still dark and one of the domestic staff was quietly waking patients with an early morning tea. I followed the tea trolley and discovered that all of the private rooms were set on the outside of a circular layout with a concourse in the centre, which housed the reception, offices and sluice rooms. Just as I was coming around the other side of the circle, I bumped into Richard the Surgeon. True to his word, he had come to check on me and to offer more words of encouragement before my operation.

At this stage in the procedure, I knew there was no going back and my resignation had an almost calming effect on me. I returned to my room and dressed myself in a surgical gown just before the porter arrived to wheel me down to the operating theatre. The journey on the trolley proved to be quite entertaining as the porter and the nurse joked with me and, before long, we were entering the pre-med room where the anaesthetist, who I had met the previous day, was preparing my anaesthetic cocktail.

He asked me how I was feeling and I was able to genuinely reassure him that I was quite calm and, although I was not looking forward to the discomfort or pain I would be in as a result of the operation, I would be pleased when the operation was over. After all there would be a positive outcome to this surgery, unlike the last major surgery I had encountered fourteen months previously, where there was a combination of positive and negative situations: the cancer had been removed but I was left breastless!

CHAPTER 23

A BABY'S HEARTBEAT?

THE whole experience in the theatre recovery room was not the least bit as harrowing as I had envisaged and my next memory of the ordeal was waking up, with a friendly nurse bending over me, fiddling with various tubes. I remember thinking that there doesn't seem to be much pain and I feel very alert. How can this be and did I really have the operation?! However, I was soon made aware of a protrusion on the front of my chest. Looking down the top of my hospital gown there were large pieces of surgical wadding held on by a gauze band. I assumed that underneath the bandages were my new breasts.

The nurse explained that, every half hour, my new breasts would be checked and, using a hand-held ultrasound detector, she would be able to ensure that the new breasts' blood supply was functioning successfully. When she pulled back the bandages protecting my chest, I avoided looking at the site of the operation, knowing that, at this early stage, it wouldn't be very pretty and, as I just wasn't ready to confront my new breasts, I averted my eyes.

Watching the nurse lean over me, I was curious to see where she placed the pen-like instrument. Gently rubbing some gel–like substance across the top of what I assumed was the newly-transplanted tissue she then moved the instrument across my chest wall.

All of a sudden I could hear a pulse just like the sound of a baby's heartbeat when a pregnant mother receives an ultrasound scan. 'Sounds good', she said and, satisfied that my new breasts were still alive and producing a strong pulse, she continued recording my blood pressure and checking my oxygen levels. I was aware of two tubes coming out of my nose and understood this to be a continuous supply of oxygen, necessary for a short time until I stabilised, following the operation, and this was probably the main reason that I felt so awake and alert.

Due to all of the tubes and the catheter attached to me, moving proved difficult and there was no way I would be going far. Shifting around in the bed was difficult, though necessary at times, as the plastic mattress cover added to the terrific sweats I was encountering. Any post-operative discomfort was initially controlled through a derivative of morphine, so I was quite comfortable in terms of managing the pain.

However, this did lull me into a false sense of well-being and, when Richard visited me, he was so surprised to see me in such good spirits. It was early evening and my good mood was enhanced not only by my husband appearing but also by Ms Sassoon also paying me a visit and saying what a success the operation had been, only taking five and half hours instead of the usual eight. My response was to emphasise that all of the success had to be down to her and her medical team's amazing expertise and dedication.

The cynics among us may say that the surgeons in the medical profession receive generous remuneration, especially if they are paid privately. Well, all I would say to those individuals is that the vast majority of surgeons deserve every penny they receive because, without their devotion and skills, I and many more women in my position certainly would not be here today, able to share our stories.

Being given intensive nursing enabled me to have twenty-four hour care and I will always be extremely grateful and humbled by the dedication and kindness shown to me by the nursing team and doctors.

During those six days, the pain and discomfort took hold and, very early on, I was offered co-dyramol, a pain killer, which I only took occasionally, in place of the morphine. Although I am not a martyr, I do seem to have quite a high pain threshold and instinctively feel that it is important, within reason, to manage your own discomfort. The body's natural production of dopamine and endorphins can be suppressed by certain painkillers and, as I believe the body is very capable of healing itself, I did not want to hinder the healing process through taking any more toxic drugs than were required.

The vivid memory I have of the first night, besides the constant interruptions every half hour for my new breasts' heartbeat being monitored, was of my body being on fire and feeling famished. I had spent a whole day and night without food and my stomach was screaming for something to eat. The night nurse very kindly found some stale cream crackers in the staff kitchen and these, plus constant sips of water, sustained me through those first hours.

The morning after the operation brought with it a new shift of friendly nursing staff, who were to carry on the intensive half-hourly monitoring. Despite the fact that I hadn't eaten much, it wasn't long before my bowels wanted to open and, as a bedpan didn't appeal to me, I asked if I could get up. The nurse seemed surprised by my request but provided me with a commode at the side of my bed.

Focusing on the commode as my goal, with every ounce of energy plus assistance from the nurse, I eased myself gingerly towards the edge of the bed. Ms Sassoon had given me strict instructions not to stand upright for at least the first week and there was no way I was able to make my torso vertical even if I had wanted to. The searing pain across my stomach was excruciating and was accompanied by the intense heat that had plagued me through the night. Little by little I edged my way onto the commode and sat, bent forward, clasping my chest and tummy.

The nurse had given me a pillow to hug as a support while I sat there for about forty minutes, determined to finish what I had started! I knew from bitter experience, when I had my hysterectomy, how important it is, following an operation, that the bowels be opened as soon as possible. The wait was worth it and the nurses who were making up my bed seemed surprised at my fortitude. There was no way I was going to give up after experiencing so much pain getting on to the mobile loo and the thought of an uncomfortable bedpan just reinforced my staying power.

As the nurses made my bed, I sensed that they were anxious for me to finish on the commode so they could complete their monitoring. There seemed to be a tight schedule to adhere to and the forthcoming rounds of Consultants' visits were putting them under pressure. To their relief, they were finally able to put me back to bed just as Ms Sassoon entered the room.

Unfortunately, much to her disgust, there hadn't been enough time to dispose of the contents of the commode. Encountering the rather unpleasant odour, Ms Sassoon threw open the window and sharply requested that the commode be taken to the sluice. She claimed that I was the first patient of hers to open the bowels so soon after the operation and, as part of post operative recovery, always recommended a daily Guinness to assist in this process!

During her examination of me, she once again reassured me that the operation had gone very well and explained that the next few days would be crucial in ensuring that the blood vessels of the transferred tissue would knit successfully to the blood vessels of the existing chest tissue. The blood supply that was pumping through the new artery running along the top of my new breasts seemed to be behaving itself and, so far, appeared to be carrying out the function for which it was intended. This was good news and, although I didn't quite feel the euphoria that a nursing sister had said some women experience, following this type of operation, I was relieved and grateful that everything had gone well.

Each day Ms Sassoon came to see me and was often accompanied by a group of Registrars all keen to study my new breasts and comment on how fine they looked. One Registrar even came back to take photographs for a seminar he was attending. I have never exposed myself to so many men in my life and probably am never likely to again!

I was pleased to cooperate if it would help in some way towards furthering medical advancements concerning the reconstruction of women's breasts, using the perforator flap technique. All of the doctors were very young, extremely professional and held Ms Sassoon in such high regard. As time went on and I watched her at work, I, too, became in awe of her exceptional talents and skills and marvelled at her attention to detail, her intuition and her tenacity. She and her team had worked a miracle on me, although I was still unable to pluck up the courage to view my new breasts and preferred to focus entirely on dealing with the recovery from my operation.

The six days I was in hospital passed by quite quickly and, once the drips and catheter were removed, I was slowly able to carry out my bodily functions, such as showering and washing my hair, independently. Showering was a slow process and required me to sit on a plastic stool, leaning forward, being careful not to wet the front of my body. I didn't care how awkward it was or how long it took as long as I could wash. Two days without a shower rendered me feeling nauseated every time I caught a whiff of the stale blood and sweat that covered my body.

A physiotherapist showed me how to move around appropriately in order to keep the pain from my wounds to a minimum. Immediately following the operation, I was painfully aware that the chest infection and cough had left me with a hideous amount of mucus. When the physiotherapist had examined me, he confirmed this and showed me the correct way to cough to bring up the phlegm and prevent my symptoms from turning into something more sinister such as pneumonia. Ms Sassoon's warning before the operation had come back to haunt me!

This coughing technique worked very effectively, the difficulty was dealing with the pain which racked my body each time a tickle appeared in my throat and I was forced to try to eject the green mucous trapped in my lungs. My life-saver proved to be in the form of a pillow, which I clung to my abdomen every time I plucked up courage to expel the substance from my throat. Fortunately, I had been given strong antibiotics, which I knew would help clear up any infections.

The day for me to be discharged soon arrived and the medical team had been pleased with the way my recovery had progressed. The transplanted 'flaps' were obviously enjoying their new home and the blood supply was well and truly established.

Ms Sassoon was still insisting that I was not to stand upright and all of my limbs were awkwardly compensating for the bent posture I was forced to adopt. This didn't worry me as I was delighted that everything had so far gone according to plan and each day I was becoming stronger.

CHAPTER 24

ANOTHER LUMP!

THE accommodation we had rented was just outside Norwich and proved to be ideal for someone who was going to be slightly disabled for a while. The two-bedroom cottage, on one level and with wonderful countryside views, was very practical and conformed to the request made by my surgeon that I wasn't to use any stairs for at least six weeks. Our experience of winter-time in Norfolk was of bright, crisp and frosty days. Watching the occasional duck on the pond in the cottage garden and the many robins was, at times, a real tonic during my recovery.

For the first week, until the pain had subsided a little and I was able to move more easily in bed, Richard and I slept in separate rooms. It wasn't necessary to interrupt Richard too much during the night to help me, as a perfect bed specifically made for the disabled had been provided in the well-equipped cottage. The bed was as effective as any hospital bed and the electrically-operated hand control moved it up and down. This helped me enormously when getting in and out of bed, which I frequently did during the night due the continuous bouts of coughing and visits to the toilet.

Once I had mastered the ability to be mobile in the cottage and made sure I was never too far away from my pillow, just in case I had another coughing fit, I pleaded with Richard to take me out for walk. My body was screaming for fresh air and my experience from the mastectomy showed me that my recovery would be even further improved if I could get my muscles and circulation working more efficiently.

Shuffling around the cottage proved to be a totally different ball game to venturing outside into the crisp January air. Trussed up like a turkey to guard against the cold, leaning heavily on Richard, I managed to walk only thirty yards before I was begging him to take me back. Disappointed, I realised that becoming mobile enough to carry out long walks in the country was going to be another lengthy process. I comforted myself with the thought that, with Richard's loving care, an organic diet full of healthy juices, my vitamin supplement protocol and plenty of sleep and rest I would soon be permanently on my feet.

We settled into a steady routine, which included two or three times daily inhaling with Olbas Oil and coughing up the never-ending mucous which stubbornly refused to leave my chest. Just as I thought the infection had cleared, a tickle would appear and I would have to hastily make for the bathroom basin and position myself on a chair clutching a pillow to support my stomach, while I coughed and spluttered, retching up what felt like the entire contents of my stomach. The moral of this part of my journey is to listen to your surgeon because mine knew the consequences of taking the risk of entering the operating theatre with a chest infection. Boy, was I learning my lesson!

It was about a week before I mustered the courage to peek at my new breasts as I was still showering with my chest covered. Every few days, I would have to change my steri-strips, which were transparent plasters which aided the healing of the scar tissue. My first impressions were favourable, and so were Richard's, and, if you looked beyond the red pulsating scarring and stitches, you would realise what a fantastic job the surgeons had achieved.

At my first weekly appointment with the plastic surgery unit, my dressings were changed and I was offered advice on the type of bra I should wear initially. Well, it proved quite a challenge to find the correct shape and material, without wires and with sufficient support. Eventually, about six bras later, I found a suitable one that did not rub my scarring too much. These shopping expeditions proved a good relationship-building exercise with my new bust and I soon realised that I was becoming quite fond of them. It was as though they had always been there!

As the days turned into weeks, I felt my body getting stronger and stronger. The concoction of antibiotics I had received, following my operation, seemed to have helped in turning my immune system around, as I certainly seemed to be keeping any infections at bay. Weekend visits from our daughter and son-in-law and our grandson, and my sister and her husband, all helped to make my convalescence pass more quickly. I religiously did as I was told by the surgeon, I made sure that I followed the exercise sheet given to me by the hospital and everything continued to heal as it should. Armed with further instructions on how to continue my good progress and an appointment for July for my nipple reconstruction, we left Stable Cottage, in some ways rather reluctantly, and headed off back to Dorset to await the arrival of our second grandchild in February.

What a wonderful surprise we had when our daughter delivered a healthy, beautiful, raven-haired daughter. Mariella is yet another angel sent to us and, like her brother, continues to make every day so special.

The May appointment with my Oncologist soon came around and we headed off to Spain. With our daughter promising to pay us a visit with her children, the time away from our wonderful grandchildren would be more bearable.

The appointment had come at a good time because a rather hard lump had appeared above my new left breast and I was convinced my Spanish Doctor would insist on some tests. I wouldn't say I was particularly worried at this stage as I felt so well. I just felt it necessary to get it checked out and I knew I was in the best possible place.

Sure enough, once the Oncologist had examined me, he advised having an ultrasound test as a precautionary measure. He, too, was confident that it was nothing to worry about and the ultrasound results suggested it was fatty tissue that had become hard.

However, he wanted a biopsy, just to be doubly sure. By this time, we had e-mailed Ms Sassoon, who insisted that it was fatty tissue, that it was nothing to worry about and that it would disperse on its own and under no circumstances was I to have a biopsy. Too late! By the time I had received her reply, a needle had been thrust into my new breast and tissue taken from the lump for analysis.

At this stage, both Richard and I became a little nervous as the memory of my first biopsy came flooding back. Richard had searched on the Internet for evidence of what the lump could be, other than the reoccurrence of the cancer and had discovered a condition called necrosis. This hardening of tissue sometimes occurs, following an operation, and often disperses in time. We held on to the belief that was the condition I had and that Ms Sassoon was right in her diagnosis.

The results would not be ready for another seven days and the total waiting time to receive a reliable diagnosis evolved into three long weeks. Meanwhile our daughter and her family arrived and occupied our days until we were to receive the results. Finally, the Oncologist was able to give us good news. The lump had turned out to be necrosis and, as a bonus, my routine blood tests showed good results.

The experience demonstrated for me that we must begin putting the whole cancer experience in perspective. After all, I really felt that I was nearing the end of the tunnel and we couldn't spend the rest of our lives constantly thinking that the cancer had returned. I was doing everything a person could do to keep healthy. I had an excellent medical team looking after me and a lot of positive energy surrounding my life and we must not forget my two new size 36B breasts. What more could I want?

The two new breasts continued to need tender loving care as the scar tissue was still very red and pulsating. Therefore, every day I massaged rosehip and vitamin E oil across the centre and underneath my breasts, not forgetting my newly positioned belly button and horizontal scar which ran across my flattened stomach, as these scars needed nurturing as well. Slowly, there was a change in the texture and colour of the scar tissue and my chest looked as though it had always housed my fine new breasts.

Psychologically, I could feel my self-esteem improving as I came to terms with, and accustomed to, my new figure. Having adjusted to having no breasts and changing my style of dress to suit the predicament, I now had to rethink my wardrobe. Although I must say it felt sensational to wear clothes that draped nicely over the bust, especially tee-shirts. I still couldn't quite pluck up courage to wear anything too low cut, but that really had never been my style anyway.

What was a whole new experience for me was buying attractive underwear. With the flat chest I had lived with previously there never seemed to be much point to spending lots of money on good quality lingerie. My standard comment had been to ask what the point was of wearing classy underwear because, if you had a good relationship, you never kept it on long enough to appreciate it anyway! How wrong can you be, and clothes shopping became even more enjoyable!

Joking aside, words cannot express my gratitude to the exceptional men and women who have been responsible and involved in the research, development and creativity during the last decade which has provided the technique of reconstructing a woman's breast, using her own tissue.

I will always be grateful to the friend who passed on to me the tabloid article about Ms Sassoon and her team. On this occasion, a British tabloid had provided some sound advice, which has hopefully benefitted many more women's lives. On reflection, the swimming experience I had in Florida was the main catalyst for my making the final decision to pursue reconstruction and, every day, I celebrate my two new breasts. I am sure Richard does too!

Chapter 25

More Operations

BUOYED up by my third six-monthly positive blood test results and with our bodies topped up with the Spanish sunshine, we returned to the UK to join in family life with our daughter and her family. Summer 2009 was very enjoyable and we spent days picnicking with the children and taking them to the park and beach.

I welcomed in the month of July as this would mean the last but one procedure to complete the look of my new breasts. It required another week-long visit to Norwich to allow the surgeon to create two nipples for me. Obviously, my original nipples had been lost when my breasts had been removed and it had been explained to me that tissue would be taken either from my earlobe or labia and grafted on to the breast to fashion new nipples. To create the effect and colour of the areola, a plastic surgery nurse would tattoo the area surrounding the new nipple, three months later.

I was not looking forward to the surgeon playing around with my genitals and had naively asked if this would affect my sex life. On hearing this question I received a retort from Ms Sassoon, pronouncing words to the effect that I shouldn't be so ridiculous and she proceeded to examine my private parts. 'No problem', was her response to the examination and, when I entered the hospital for the day procedure I was convinced I would be going home with two fine nipples but unable to sit down!

How relieved was I when I sat on the edge of the hospital bed on the morning of the surgery to hear that Ms Sassoon had decided to use an envelope of redundant skin which fortunately was part of the scar tissue in the crease of my new right breast. Not only would the procedure be more comfortable for me but I was sure it would be more straightforward for the surgeon.

We had rented another country property for the week to enable me to attend the first check up, following the skin graft, and to have peace and quiet to aid recovery. It had also been decided that I required a little more tissue to be added to the upper part of my left breast to make them both more uniform. Therefore, a second procedure was booked in for the following week.

It was early morning as I walked down to theatre and I wasn't too nervous as I had been reassured by the fact that it was to be carried out under local anaesthetic. I had assumed this would mean not much pain and discomfort and I was quite looking forward to seeing how my new nipples would look. As usual the nursing staff were lovely and attempted to put me at ease, instructing me to place my hands behind my back as they sterilised me with a cold solution.

I lay there wondering how I would be able to keep still for the required hour or so, as I am such a fidget, and hoping that my arms wouldn't go to sleep due to the position I was in. Ms Sassoon appeared and immediately the room seemed to quieten, fewer jokes were made and I tried to break the tension by asking a couple of questions about the operation.

As the responses were rather curt, I, too, fell silent and only spoke when spoken to - quite a feat for me! The local anaesthetic kicked in and, although I was conscious of the surgeon cutting underneath my right breast, I tried not to think about what was happening to me. As she worked away at transferring the small pieces of skin to the centre of my breast and fashioning them into nipples I likened the whole experience to attending the dentist when you have a tooth pulled. You are aware of what is happening and, although there is no real pain due to the area being numb, you are conscious that something rather uncomfortable is taking place.

As the surgeon skilfully tugs and pulls and finally cuts the area, it is better if you transfer your thoughts to a far away place and not dwell too much on what is happening to you. Well, that's how I got through the whole hour and half, lying on my back, staring at bright, coloured theatre lights, thinking pleasant thoughts and reliving happy moments with my grandchildren.

It was soon all over and, after a cup of tea and a sandwich, I was discharged with the instructions not to take my bandages off as they would be removed when I returned to the hospital the following Monday. Disappointed that I would not be seeing my new nipples for another week, I comforted myself with the fact that I did not seem to be in much pain.

When I examined the bandaging that was taped all around my chest the shape of my breasts had changed. Positioned where I presumed my new nipples would be was an egg box cone shape, which had a spongy texture. The cone had a flat top so, under clothes, my breasts looked a strange flattened pyramid shape. All week, I wore a gilet to try to disguise the misshapen protrusions.

Added to this, showering proved very difficult. I resorted to sitting in the bath, trying desperately not to wet the front of my body. Around day five, I was desperate to wash my hair and I had a brainwave to strap bin liners around my chest to make the bandages waterproof. Big mistake!

As I stood in the shower, enjoying the sensation of being able to wet my hair I soon felt the water running down the inside of the plastic sheeting. Quickly finishing my shower, I attempted to rip off the protective cover and, to my horror, and not surprisingly, the bandage came off as well. Quick action was required to decide how I was going to rebandage myself, as we realised that the foam protective cups would not stay on my breasts by themselves.

Well, at last I caught a peek at my nipples, which I must say looked incredibly scabby and red and not very impressive. However, experience had taught me that if the skin graft had taken, and sometimes they do fail, the nipples' appearance would improve with time. Therefore, all I could think about was drying out the gauze.

Using a hairdryer would have been a good option but unfortunately we had forgotten to bring one. Therefore, I resorted to standing in front of the oven hoping this would at least dry me out enough to use some sticking plaster and tape it all back together. Fortunately there were only two days to go before I would be back at the hospital and it would be removed. I never dreamed that my stupid mistake would bring the wrath of my surgeon down on my head.

Once more, I found myself heading for the hospital for my second operation at the mercy of Ms Sassoon, of whom, I might add, I had become very fond, and enjoyed her unusual bedside manner. We always managed to have a little banter and, although she had only met me about five times for about thirty minutes each time, putting aside the time on the operating table, I felt she was instinctively getting to know me quite well.

It was to my detriment that, when I found myself sitting on the bed awaiting an escort to theatre, I fully realised how intuitive she was and how much she had come to know my little idiosyncrasies. When she discovered that my dressings had become wet and had been removed, she was not pleased. Explaining to me that within each of the protective cups there had been a special substance to encourage healing, she proceeded to scold me about how it would have been a good idea to have returned to the hospital where they would have redressed my wounds. I sat there like a naughty little school girl, in silence, unable to defend myself. I had not fully appreciated that I was within my rights to contact the hospital and have the area redressed. Richard said he was so shocked as to how well I took her reprimand on the chin.

This was so not my style, always being at the forefront of something to say and questioning everything. It was seven-thirty in the morning. What with still feeling half asleep, a little nervous about the next operation and knowing that Ms Sassoon was right, I decided to defer to her authority. She turned to Richard and enquired as to whether I was always so disobedient as she had come to the conclusion that I didn't very often do as I was told. Smiling Richard agreed and between them they had a little joke about how Richard had never before seen me stumped for words. I did not object to being teased as I just wanted my surgeon to be in a good temper when I was on the operating table! She left to prepare for the surgery and it wasn't long before I found myself being prepared for yet another operation.

The nurses remembered me from the previous week and, after the standard ice-breaking welcomes, chuckling,

I explained how I was in Ms Sassoon's bad books. I could tell from her eyes that she wasn't really harbouring any grudge as a result of me misbehaving and, before she got down to business, we even managed to have an interesting conversation about her beloved cat, 'Pimms'.

Whilst my body was being sterilised, I was introduced to a friendly, younger nurse who explained that she would be sitting with me throughout the operation. We had a pleasant chat during the surgery and I was able to ask her questions about the procedure.

It wasn't until much later on, having experienced this strange technique, that I realised precisely the reason I had been allocated a nurse to sit alongside me. The objective of the treatment was to remove some fat from my inner thigh and transfer it to the upper part of my left breast. This additional padding of fat would fill in a small indentation, allowing my left breast to be rounded, fuller and more uniform with my right - a straightforward task, or so I had thought.

I don't wish to sound complacent or blasé and I knew nothing would ever be as uncomfortable as the major reconstruction operation I had had in January, or my bi-lateral mastectomy, but I really did imagine that taking a little fat from my rather wobbly thigh would not cause too much discomfort. I even joked about whether Ms Sassoon would mind sorting out all my areas of cellulite.

Completely pain free, I was conscious of work being carried out on my inner right thigh. With digging sensations and lots of crunching sounds, I followed the movements of the surgeon as best I could whilst lying on my arms, which were behind my back. Sam, the 'patient-sitting' nurse, tried her best to take my mind off what was happening by asking me questions about my family. Unexpectedly, she heard how we had three children, the eldest had died and now we had two beautiful grandchildren. (If questioned about my family I always make reference to John, not ever wanting to deny his existence).

I quickly moved away from family matters and on to the subject in hand, as the surgeon and her assistant were standing away from my body and were focusing on a rather strange looking tube like structure which was making a noise. Relieved that they appeared to have finished with my thigh, I wanted to know what they were doing. Nurse Sam proceeded to explain that having used a large syringe-type instrument to remove the fat, it was now necessary to spin it until it solidified like lard. Once this part of the procedure was completed the hardened fat would be pumped into my chest wall.

After what seemed like an age Ms Sassoon used an injection to numb the left side of my chest area in preparation for the installation of the 'filler fat'. This implant of fat proved to be a very weird sensation indeed and at one point I experienced an uncomfortable ramming feeling as though the instrument being used to install the fat was coming through my chest wall. It seemed that it was necessary for the surgeon to push the fat as far into the new breast as possible to ensure that it became embedded well into its new home. Further local anaesthetic was used to ensure I remained as comfortable as possible and I was certainly glad when the process was completed.

A couple of hours later I was discharged from hospital with a stern warning from Ms Sassoon not to do too much and she also obtained reassurance from Richard that he would keep a close watch on me. It was important that the new fat was not absorbed by the body and remained just where it had been installed and served its function of shaping the top half of my left breast.

Driving back to the cottage, I described to Richard the whole process and made a firm decision that I would do as I was told as I had no intention of repeating that particular experience if the new fat dispersed.

Over the next few days I was rather weepy and my mood was, surprisingly, a little low. Blaming the residual effects of the local anaesthetic, I took long walks in the fresh Norfolk air and rested when I needed to. The most painful area, following the small liposuction surgery, was the large bruised area on my leg where the fat had been removed and for the first couple of days I had difficulty walking.

Reflecting on the whole in-filling process, I could now appreciate what it must be like to have liposuction as well as a tummy tuck. All I will say is that if I had been in the position of having the choice to have these two types of procedure, simply because of vanity, I would have declined. Individuals who put themselves through any cosmetic surgery, simply as way of holding back the years, are either very brave or very stupid because it is certainly not pain free.

I was fortunate to have two of the best plastic surgeons and their teams in the country, if not the world, which gave me the confidence to go through with the procedure. However, there were still many moments when I was scared, in chronic pain and wondering whether I was doing the right thing.

Each to their own, but there will be no more cosmetic surgery for me. I just want to grow old gracefully and healthily.

As we travelled back to Bournemouth, it was a marvellous feeling to think that nearly all of the operating procedures were behind me. One more visit to Norfolk remained, for an appointment to have two areolas tattooed around my new nipples, and then the reconstruction process would be completed.

We had always strongly advised our children never to have a tattoo and I hoped they wouldn't see their mother as too much of a hypocrite!

The whole tattoo experience proved to be quite straightforward, only taking about half an hour and was carried out by one of the breast care nurses who had been trained in the specialist procedure. Once she had carefully drawn a mark around the new nipples to indicate where the new areolas were to be tattooed, the nurse and I chose the appropriate coloured dye to match my skin tone. In fact, two colours were mixed together and, fortunately, the ink is made up of natural additives. It is applied using a special tattooing needle and the overall effect is created using a series of injections all radiating from the needle. Once the procedure was completed, I was told to apply Vaseline to the tattoo twice a day and was then allowed to go home. A slight redness and scabs appeared around the tattoo area which, apparently, was quite normal and only lasted a couple of days. After about a year, the tattoos would fade and I was entitled to return to the clinic for a tattoo touch-up but, to date, I haven't felt the need to do this because they still look very authentic. In fact, the slight fading helps the area to blend more realistically with my existing skin colour.

The whole tattoo procedure provided the icing on the cake as far as my new breasts were concerned and, at last, I really was feeling that they had always been a part of me. In fact, I have forgotten what the old breasts looked like!

CHAPTER 26

THE END OF THE JOURNEY?

THE main reason for opening this self-help book with such a tragic story is to explain that I believe that we are not here by chance but that we are all travelling our own unique journey and that being diagnosed with breast cancer has given me the opportunity to put into perspective the purpose of my journey. It has provided an opportunity for you, the reader, to share the events of this period of my life with me and acquire some useful information that may help you, your loved ones and anyone else who may or may not be experiencing the journey through cancer.

Generally, I have tried to describe my journey with candour and at times with a little humour. However, although there were many occasions when I was frightened and anxious for myself and my family, at no time did I ever feel like giving up. At the beginning of my journey, the light at the end of the tunnel appeared dim but, as the weeks went by and my body became fitter and my hair thicker and curlier, the light became stronger and my resolve improved.

Christmas 2009 proved to be a very different one from the one we had spent the previous year. Joining our son in Qatar, who provided us with a delightful family Christmas, and spending lazy days on the beach, eating good food and enjoying rounds of golf and party games all proved to be just what the doctor ordered. The pleasure of seeing our eighteen-month old grandchild opening his Christmas presents, playing with his uncle on the beach and swimming in the pool reinforced the sweetness of family life.

The turning point came as I reached the end of the tunnel in March 2009, exactly thirteen months after my chemotherapy. One day I was suddenly aware that I felt incredibly well and the heaviness that pervaded my body had lifted and it no longer dragged itself around, almost waiting for the next infection to manifest itself.

It was two months since my January operation and everyone had told me that the recovery I had made was incredible. One reason for the sudden turn around in my health, I am sure, was due to the antibiotics that had been administered to me in hospital and I instinctively felt that they had mopped up a number of viruses lurking in my blood. Secondly, I had restarted my supplement protocol two months earlier, after stopping it on the advice from my surgeon, just before the breast reconstruction procedures and the regime was, once more, having a positive effect. Thirdly, the chemotherapy was now becoming a distant bad dream with the complex cellular structure of my body increasingly feeling the relief of the passage of time over the past thirteen months. It was obvious this was being borne out in the guise of my stronger constitution.

The progress I had made was also confirmed when I had my six-monthly check up in Spain, with my blood test, for the first time, showing the results of each component of my blood being in the appropriate range. I was thrilled and my confidence was boosted even further when poor Richard appeared to go down with the flu rather badly and

I managed to escape the same fate.

I returned to running to try to combat the excess weight that had accumulated since I had starting taking the Tamoxifen and had been more sedentary following my January operation. During the time I took Tamoxifen, it was tolerable, and I did not seem to suffer too much with the usual day-to-day side effects such as hot flushes, although I did notice that, if I failed to exercise, my legs became rather bloated.

Taking the anti-oestrogen drug for five years is the recommended timescale and, although I understood the relevance of reducing my oestrogen levels, thus starving the oestrogen dependant breast cancer that I had, I was concerned about the long-term side effects. When I expressed my worries about the long term effects and suggested that maybe I could abstain from the drug, my oncologist was adamant that to stop taking it wasn't an option. My family were also very against me giving it up and, therefore, Tamoxifen stayed in my life for three years. (I was then moved on to another aromatase inhibitor, Exemestane, which can be taken as an alternative medication to Tamoxifen, and remained on this for a further two years, again with few side effects).

Reaching the end of the tunnel that had been such a part of my life for nearly two years was a welcome relief and there were many days where the previous months seemed to have happened to someone else. There was just the occasional moment when I remembered the nauseating experience of the chemotherapy, the pain of my operations or fear when sharing the diagnosis with family and friends. Common sense told me that this was all part of the letting-go process and, just as my body had taken time to recover, so would my mind. However, these moments were becoming fewer and fewer and I was even managing to read about other cancer patients' stories and watch documentaries on the television, whereas, previously, I had shied away from such subjects.

Feeling so well and having two new breasts gave me a new lease of life. Spending time with our two gorgeous grandchildren was the icing on the cake and the only reminder I had of my journey through cancer was my six-monthly checkups. The October 2009 check up soon came around and, during the visit to Spain, we combined a 'well woman' and a 'well man' annual check up with the GP that we had used over the past twelve years. The routine blood test, which isn't as comprehensive as the blood test the oncologist carries out, showed I was slightly anaemic and I was immediately advised to take Folic acid and vitamin B12. Vitamin B12 is naturally found in animal products, including fish, meat, poultry, eggs, milk, and milk products. However, it is generally not present in plant foods and, therefore, if you are a vegetarian, it is a very important to take a supplement of the B12 vitamin, preferably the complete B complex. The doctor wasn't unduly worried as I had had a history of slight anaemia on and off since 2003.

I was not surprised at the results as I had felt a little more tired than usual and I had blamed it on the Spanish heat. More significantly I had stopped taking my 'B' complex because I had recently reviewed our vitamin protocol with the objective of trying to cut down the amount of supplements we were consuming. Feeling confident that our fresh organic diet was extremely nourishing, I had wrongly assumed that this was the group of vitamins we could manage without. Situations such as these show me that I must never become complacent about my health and

I will always ensure that my health protocol is a high priority in my life and review it periodically.

Interestingly enough, one week before my check-up with the GP in Spain, I had noticed an advertisement about a vitamin test as part of an iridology consultation. Instinctively, I followed it up and was pleased to discover that I was only lacking in a couple of health components, 'B' vitamins being one of them. Coincidently the blood test taken later confirmed this and I am now even more convinced that many alternative tests such as allergy checking and the iridology process are very useful backups to the more standard medical blood tests. If the therapist is well-trained they are able to offer advice and recommendations on the patient's protocol which often a GP is not qualified or experienced enough to do.

The iridology report showed a possible lymphatic congestion throughout my body, an inflamed digestive tract and a need for a general detox. Once again, I had listened to my body and instinctively knew that my whole system was feeling extremely sluggish, which had been confirmed by the iridology investigation.

Fortunately, as soon as we had arrived in Spain, I had commenced a programme of lymphatic drainage. Using a previous contact who was able to perform deep-tissue massage, the benefits were felt immediately and, suffering more than usual with indigestion and heartburn, I included digestive enzymes and pro-biotic supplements into my protocol. Although I was very fortunate that nearly two years on, the Lymphoedema condition had not yet presented itself and my right arm appeared to be as strong as my left, I was aware that, medically speaking, the removal of fourteen Lymph nodes would mean that my body's lymphatic system would always be impaired.

The liver, a large component of the lymph system, would probably be still in recovery from a toxic overload due to the chemotherapy drugs and the Tamoxifen would also be a contributing factor to this overload.

Originally, following the mastectomy, my right arm had often felt heavy and swollen and I was concerned that these symptoms were manifesting themselves into lymphoedema. However, since my breast reconstruction operation ten months previously, I had noticed that all of the previous symptoms had disappeared. A discussion I had with the reconstruction surgeon revealed that, possibly, the transfer of the stomach tissue's stem cells had aided the circulation and blood flow of the area. She also mentioned something else about stem cells which I didn't understand and, not wanting to bother her further, I satisfied myself with the belief that it was yet another benefit of the marvellous surgery I had undergone.

Reflecting, during my journey, coming to terms with the fears of cancer and deciding whether this really is the end of my journey through cancer, have been some of the most important elements of my recovery.

Chapter 27

Reflections

THROUGHOUT the first year of my journey, a nagging question often raised its head. On diagnosis, I had asked the three medical specialists who were involved in my orthodox treatment: the Spanish Surgeon who removed the tumour, the UK Consultant whom I had visited for a second opinion and my Spanish Oncologist why there was no alternative cure for cancer being administered other than chemotherapy or radiotherapy?'

Not one of the specialists was able to give me a satisfactory answer and, although I had offered up my body to the care of these professionals and trusted in and was grateful for their individual expertise, the unease I felt about their approach being the only road to travel in the cure for my cancer grew at an alarming rate, thus encountering yet another paradox in my journey.

At times I felt that the medical profession seemed to be stuck in a time warp. It appeared that, in principle, the same approach for the treatment of the majority of cancers had been used since the war. It is unfair to say that there are no other orthodox approaches being trialled and extensive research and testing is being carried out as I write this book. However, as stated on the website of the US National Institute of Health (www.cancer.gov), the FDA (Food and Drug Administration) claims that the whole process of approving a new cancer drug can take on average 8.5 years! The majority of cancer patients have neither the time nor the energy to wait for the latest wonder drug and, often, they are unable to access this medication. Another consideration is the myriad of side effects that nearly always accompanies the administration of such orthodox drugs.

At the time, I pacified myself with the knowledge that I would use my own skills and research experience to discover the appropriate path for me to follow to restore myself to optimum health, ensuring that cancer would never again join me on my journey through life.

This was definitely one experience I did not want to repeat and I was determined to take the lessons I was rapidly learning about myself and use them proactively along the road to a contented healthy lifestyle in order to help myself and, perhaps, help other people along the way.

It soon became evident, as the months passed, that my desire to be as proactive as possible and ensure that my cancer experience was a learning opportunity for myself and others would lead me to discover how unpredictable the restoration of one's own body is when it has been subjected to cancer, major surgery and chemotherapy. I would need patience and could not expect to feel one hundred per cent fit immediately.

On reflection of the action I took and of all of the reading material that I assimilated during my journey, the approach to restoring my health can best be viewed as containing three components: a diagnostic health review, a nutritional plan, and a spiritual path. These aspects of restoration of my well–being were delivered alongside both the medical protocol that had been designed for me by my oncologist and a complementary health protocol, using the expertise of knowledgeable therapists. I cannot deny that the amazing equation of health restoration is enhanced by using the diagnostic abilities and expertise of the scientific and medical field.

Obviously, there needs to be an analytical approach to identify how far the disease has progressed and not just rely on hope that the health of the individual can be turned around, which is often the case with the holistic alternative. Therefore, incorporating the orthodox expertise, using the drugs that were and are available, was extremely important during my own health restoration approach.

The second vital component was to use a holistic, organic tactic. 'You Are What You Eat' became my mantra during the journey to restoring my diseased body to health. During the chemotherapy, my practically vegan diet was enhanced with supplements of vitamins, minerals, herbs and spices.

The nutritional approach to my cancer protocol was not a difficult concept to comprehend, but to administer this approach required a great deal of understanding about which foods contain which restorative qualities. It is, therefore, understandable that the majority of doctors in the medical profession are not trained in the nutritional field and, therefore, will sometimes only offer the occasional piece of advice on what and why we should eat certain nutrients.

As I was discovering that there are numerous complementary practitioners available on the Internet, in books and within one's own town or city, waiting to flood the recipients with information on the benefits of a good diet or what vita-nutrients can do to enhance one's health, it is important when using the nutritional component to seek out as much expertise as you are able to through reading, using the internet and contacting qualified nutritionists.

Throughout my journey I have never strayed too far from the view that my life force needs to be spiritually nurtured and instinctively know that the road to good health requires consideration to be given to this area, hence my involvement in the EFT therapy and yoga-breathing techniques. Cleansing from the inside was also a primary consideration using deep-lymph massage and colonic irrigation.

I often visualize my body in the centre of a circle surrounded by spiritual, emotional and physiological waves that cannot be easily separated. All are of equal importance as they blend together, ebbing and flowing backwards and forwards, ensuring the balance of the circle will not be thrown off course. However, as is too often the case, a life-changing event or unusual circumstances will occur and may break the circle of good health.

Improving the equilibrium between my spiritual self and physical health, using quality nutritional input and fine-tuning my emotional well-being was, at the time, the path to follow. I believed that I needed to counteract the interruption to this equilibrium that had been caused due to the dis-ease ebbing into my circle of life. Through learning to combine these self-help strategies in my restorative health protocol, I was beginning to understand how I was in control of improving the fine balance of my well-being. I believe that constantly behaving in a too ethereal manner or too scientific/logical or playing havoc with the nutritional side of our health only causes a disturbance in the body's equilibrium.

Therefore, the third component of my healing process was to allow my spiritual side which encompassed my view of God to enter my life once again. Through praying that the Universe's healing powers and positive energy would flood my body and ensure that the cancer was eradicated for ever had worked for me and was the journey I am glad I decided to take.

If the sphere of good health which should encompass our body is damaged and disease takes us by surprise, it is comforting to know that we can proactively help the healing through addressing the three components of the circle. Throughout the majority of my recovery period I was totally committed to every aspect of this approach. However, when doubts crept in as to whether my strategy was working and moments of sheer desperation occurred, I knew I had no choice but to travel this path. I adopted the stance that I had nothing to lose and, by being proactive, at least I was helping myself.

The trials and errors I discovered during my journey were numerous and, at times, I felt that I would give up as the obstacles placed before me seemed to be insurmountable. This is not helped when you are battling the weakness and demotivation you feel when you are undergoing chemotherapy. There are often periods of confusion when you are faced with hundreds of complementary treatments to cancer and the most difficult part of the road was attaining the medical profession's understanding and acceptance of the need to integrate natural remedies alongside the orthodox approach.

Although I consulted all of the four orthodox medical experts that I was involved with about various substances I would be taking to alleviate any side effects from the cancer drugs, the response was generally one of disinterest and a laissez-faire attitude. Naturally, I would have preferred their approval of what I was doing but I soon came to accept that showing any commitment to the complementary treatment I was undergoing may have shown an undermining of their own profession. After all, there is no denying that much of today's current medications have contributed to the healing of millions of individuals and the prevention of the spread of many contagious diseases.

However, the Spanish doctors were the most receptive of all of the medical professionals that I consulted on my journey. It is evident that there is still a long way to go before there is true integration between the medical and the alternative or complementary health practitioners and total harmony will require a change of attitudes, a shedding of suspicion and a sharing of expertise on both sides.

One fundamental difference between the complementary approach and the orthodox road to healing is that, generally, the complementary way involves looking at the whole person whilst the medical profession tends to look only at the physiology.

How many times in our everyday life do we ever contemplate the interconnectedness of our physical, emotional and spiritual wellbeing? There is a significant market of valuable information currently available that suggests how to improve each of the above aspects but rarely do we address all of them at the same time.

Trusting in your medical practitioner and finding one

who is open and who will listen to your questions and respect what might appear to them to be an unorthodox protocol will be essential to the success of your health strategy. Overcoming the illness is the main objective and it is important that all of the therapists involved in the treatment are fully aware of the treatment path being followed, especially the medical professional who is likely to be overseeing your primary care.

There may also be others involved in the care of the cancer patient and it is vital that all of the information related to the delivery of the protocol is shared and communicated clearly to ensure that the objective of improving the health and well-being of the patient is fulfilled. A positive mental attitude should be demonstrated at all times by those involved in the treatments.

During my research I came across the following succinct views from an American Doctor, Dr. Lindsey Duncan (www.genesistoday.com)

'There are very few cancer victims (although some children are victims of cancer) but by far, the majority of cancer is earned by us (you and me). Our choices and our lifestyle cause an effect. There is something I call the cancer spiral and this is how it works. The fear deep inside of us creates anger and the anger creates stress. The anger, fear and stress all feed off of ignorance. The ignorance then facilitates poor choices. The poor choices then manifest themselves in our lifestyle; diet, habits, addictions, bad relationships, stressful jobs, toxic elements, and negative thoughts, emotions, etc. All of these negative components feed off of each other and over time break down our cells, tissues, organs, bodies, minds and spirit. We wake up one day and we've earned cancer. Stop this spiral and you stop

the negative cycle that is happening everywhere around you. Change the world by changing yourself first.

'My second thought is that the cancer patient does not need fear, a death sentence, a prescription of death or to be treated as a statistic. They do, however, desperately need love, hope, a road map to health, a plan of attack, guidance, coaching, real answers, support, a teacher, a doctor, a healer, a spiritual counsellor and most importantly, they must be the lead participant. Our job as a doctor is to create this beautiful fertile ground for the lead participant.

'My final thought: don't earn cancer - do something about it now so you do not read an article like this from a cancer patient's perspective. Preventative medicine is much preferred over reactive medicine or any other medicine for that matter. An ounce of prevention really and truly is worth a ton of cure. And please remember, what we build our homes (temple) with today, will determine how we weather the storms of tomorrow.'

The above words just about sum up for me what I have felt throughout my journey, that cancer need not be feared if we take responsibility for our own health, work with our doctors and therapists and don't take anything for granted. Questioning every aspect of the journey and reflecting and researching into ways I could help myself and my healers to ensure I had the best chance of survival were my paramount objectives during my journey. With the right input, the body, this amazing complex machine, can heal itself. We just have to have the belief and the positive energy to make it happen.

Dr. Duncan's comment: 'There are very few cancer victims (although some children are victims of cancer) but by far, the majority of cancer is earned by us (you and me). Our choices and our lifestyle cause an effect' has assisted me in this reflexion period and in understanding why I have had to make this journey through cancer and arrived at this crossroads in my life.

Not appreciating the repercussions of a pretty stressful fifty-plus years and always believing that I had taken on board and dealt with all of the traumas life had thrown at me, I now realise it is not what you have to deal with, it is how you deal with it. After all, in the grand scheme of things, most people have had difficult childhoods or marriages, money worries, stressful careers, lost loved ones through tragic circumstances or natural causes and don't necessarily 'earn' cancer. In other parts of the world, we know that people are suffering far worse fates such as famine, war and disease, and never receive basic human rights. Do they 'earn' cancer? It would be very interesting to know if there are any studies carried out on the subject of cancer rates in underprivileged countries.

The death of my beloved son in 1990, and then in 2006, in close succession, my best friend's son, whom I had known all his life, and the deaths of two very close and dear friends, proved more difficult for me to deal with than I have ever admitted. Soldiering on was the only option for me and I can't say that it was all about putting on a brave face as I truly believed I had come to terms with my son's death. I now know that was not the case and another hard lesson was felt when my godson, Oliver, died.

On reflection, the grief I had felt following Oliver's death was compounded by losing my two friends and the abyss that I had felt when John died engulfed me yet again and, I believe, finally manifested itself into my illness. This is not the whole story and, as I have tried to express at the beginning of this chapter of Reflections, the balance of one's mind and body are interconnected. I will never know for certain. I can only go with my instinct that I 'earned' cancer through not always looking after my mind and body.

In 2004, I trained very hard for the 2005 London Marathon, not wanting to let down the many sponsors that had supported me in my objective to raise money for the Parkinson's Society. I believe that overtraining compromised my immune system. Towards the end of my training, especially when I went out on my long runs, I would go down with runner's diarrhoea. Apparently one in four runners suffer with this condition and it can be very debilitating. The situation became so severe at one stage that I was badly anaemic and, three weeks before the race, I was given Vitamin B injections by my GP. I don't believe my body recovered properly and the diet I followed may have fallen short at times as I listened to the low-salt and low-fat advocates.

On reflection, I may not always have ingested enough of the right fats, and salt was always a no-no. There is much reliable research and information that demonstrates that many women who suffer with breast cancer are very often iodine deficient. It is a fact that today's diet is heavily laden with poor quality salt which contains little or no iodine. Nowadays, I use only a good quality sea salt which is organic and free from pollutants. The correct balance of omega and fish oils is also essential in maintaining our health and, throughout my menopausal period, I have noticed from time to time how dry my skin and hair become. My new health protocol ensures that I now rarely subject my body to unreliable foodstuffs and I will always review my diet from time to time to ensure I stay on the right track.

The Spiritual side of my philosophical circle is still being worked on and it would be very arrogant of me to say that I have arrived spiritually. It is an ongoing process of analysing one's thoughts, daily behaviour towards others and searching for inner peace and contentment. My own Christian beliefs assist me in this and my ambition, one day, is to master Meditation.

Eighteen months on and, in this period of reflection, I am trying to understand, come to terms with and decide whether this really is the end of my journey through cancer. I reflect on how the experience has affected my dear husband, children, extended family and friends. For a long period, I noticed our daughter, despite the fact she has given birth to two babies, appeared very resentful of what had happened to me. She doesn't suffer fools gladly and appeared to have little patience with many people.

Understandably, I sense there is always the fear that her mother may become ill again and she never wants us to be apart for too long. However, I am sure these changes will settle down and, with time, she will trust in life again. The whole experience has helped her to mature into a confident, dependable woman and a very competent, loving mother. We have become even closer, if that was possible. I cherish her wisdom and the support and advice she often offers me.

Our son has not talked much about his feelings concerning me contracting cancer and, living so far away from us, it has often been difficult to discuss his concerns. Thank goodness, he has a supportive wife and a strong bond with his sister. The unconditional love we have for one another is often expressed by him through his actions. Not many days pass without him contacting us and, if we needed him, he would be on the next available plane back to the UK. He is a good example of action speaking louder than words!

The only comment he made to me when I enquired of him as to how he was feeling about me having cancer certainly summed up his fears: 'Well you don't have it now do you?' He naturally wants everything to go back to being the way it was and so does my husband, if he is honest. When asked, Richard shared his reflections with me. Without a doubt, he cherishes his family and appreciates his friends much more. He says he is not so complacent about life and has faced his own mortality. Fear of what the future holds sometimes engulfs him as he anticipates the results of my six-monthly check ups. His confidence in forward planning our future has taken a knock and he is a little resentful of the dramatic change in our lifestyle with health taking more of a priority.

All of these concerns are understandable and at least the strength of our marriage enables us to talk about them and, at different times, offer comfort and reassurance. Out of the ashes of this particular journey together, I have discovered an amazing partner who has never faulted in his demonstration of his love for me and I adore him more and more each day.

Yes, I still get days and moments when I am scared that the cancer may return. They usually happen when I am feeling below par but those times are becoming less frequent. The most successful strategy I have for dealing with these doubts is to remind myself that I have the experience and knowledge, if I deem it necessary, to find out what is wrong with me and, alongside the medical profession, to draw up a protocol to put it right.

There are many proactive elements to my life now to ensure I remain healthy: I relish the love of my family, I try not to become overtired or too stressed and I drink very little alcohol. I periodically detox through increasing the number of times a day I have fresh juices or find a good quality detoxifying substance and there are plenty on the market. I ensure, wherever possible, that I eat organic food, eat fish at least three times a week and white meat once. I review my vita-nutrient regime and adjust it according to my needs. Exercise for a least an hour every day, mainly through walking or running, is essential, as are my deep lymphatic massages. I avoid wasting time with people I would rather not be around, and try to let go and not dwell on any worries that may crop up.

I have yet to meet anyone with a crystal ball, which will allow me to see what the future holds for myself and my family, and I am glad I haven't. I enjoy the moment, look forward to the future with excitement and enthusiasm and remember the words of my wonderful mother, who following her horrendous divorce in 1969, told me that what kept her going, besides her children, was to look ahead. She also described how she felt about life and, considering the many worries she had with her family, I never cease to be amazed at how she never became too bitter. Offering another benefit of her wisdom, right up until the final days of her life (she passed away in April, 2013), she looked forward every night, when she went to bed, to the pleasures the next day may bring.

The journey through cancer has shown me many paradoxes, some of which I have outlined in this journey. However, the main paradox for me has been that, out of the initial fear that invades anyone who is diagnosed with cancer, has emerged a new-found freedom. A freedom from the fear of cancer because I know that I have learnt so many valuable lessons about my inner self and my physical health and I am still continuing to learn. Being empowered with a degree of knowledge acquired through actually experiencing the disease has enabled me to write this book and, hopefully, other people may benefit from my experience. Out of the fear has grown a certain enrichment of life and the confidence that I can help my body to turn my health around if necessary.

For all the negatives such a disease ushers in, there are positive aspects too. One such positive is my ability to be more empathetic with others without behaving as I always did by being a 'people pleaser'. Without a doubt, the cancer has changed me as a person. In fact, it has changed many people around me. However, the experiences I have encountered in my journey through cancer are still too close to reflect on how much I have changed and I am still getting to know the new me. One thing I am aware of is that the journey through cancer has come to an end and my journey through life can now continue with the same degree of excitement that has always been part of my life force.

ABOUT THE AUTHOR

CATH FILBY was born in Newport, Wales in 1954. She trained and worked in banking when she left school and then, married with three children, changed career and worked in vocational training. Later, Cath with her husband of 41 years, ran a highly successful national training organisation for twelve years.

Following the death of her son in 1990, Cath and her husband took early retirement in 1998, and went to live in Southern Spain, where they enjoyed an idyllic existence until her life was shattered by the diagnosis of Breast Cancer in 2007. The experiences she encountered on her journey through cancer inspired her to write her memoirs and design a self-help health book, which she hopes will inspire others to take control of their lives during their journeys through cancer.

When they are not busy writing and travelling, Cath and her husband spend quality family time with their children and grandchildren in Qatar and Australia.

ENJOYED
THIS BOOK? WE'VE GOT LOTS MORE!

BRITAINSNEXTBESTSELLER.CO.UK

Britain's Next
BESTSELLER

DISCOVER NEW INDEPENDENT BOOKS & HELP AUTHORS GET A PUBLISHING DEAL.

DECIDE WHAT BOOKS WE PUBLISH NEXT & MAKE AN AUTHOR'S DREAM COME TRUE.

Visit **www.britainsnextbestseller.co.uk** to view book trailers, read book extracts, pre-order new titles and get exclusive Britain's Next Bestseller Supporter perks.

FOLLOW US:

 BNBSbooks   @bnbsbooks   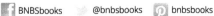 bnbsbooks